THE OFFICIAL

booty parlor ®

MOJO

MAKEOVER

Four Weeks to a Sexier You

DANA B. MYERS

HARPER

HarperCollins books may be purchased for educational,
business, or sales promotional use. For information
please write: Special Markets Department, HarperCollins
Publishers, 10 East 53rd Street, New York, NY 10022.

FIRST EDITION

Designed by Janet M. Evans

Library of Congress Cataloging-in-Publication Data is
available upon request.

ISBN 978-0-06-198744-1

11 12 13 14 15   OV/QGF   10 9 8 7 6 5 4 3 2

To all my Booty Parlor babes.
You helped shape this makeover
by sharing
your secrets, your desires,
and your experiences with me . . .
and you're walking proof
that confidence is sexy!

CONTENTS

INTRODUCTION
YOU, ME, AND THE
MOJO MAKEOVER
viii

CHAPTER ONE
Introducing the Mojo Makeover
3

CHAPTER TWO
The Mojo Makeover Questionnaire
14

CHAPTER THREE
What Hinders Your Mojo
32

WEEK ONE: CLEAN OUT YOUR
SEXUAL CLOSET
45

CHAPTER FOUR
*Give Your Wardrobe a
Mojo Makeover*
46

CHAPTER FIVE
*Turning Mojo Malfunctions
into Mojo Musts*
54

CHAPTER SIX
*Creating Seductive Beauty
and Body Rituals*
67

WEEK TWO: INFUSE
EVERY DAY
WITH SEX APPEAL
87

CHAPTER SEVEN
Let's Talk About Sex, Girls!
88

CHAPTER EIGHT
Sexy-up Your Wardrobe
99

CHAPTER NINE
Make Over Your Bedroom
113

WEEK THREE: HAVE
THE SEX YOU NEED—
AND DESERVE
121

CHAPTER TEN
Communicate Your Desires
122

CHAPTER ELEVEN

The Big 5-O Program

131

CHAPTER TWELVE

Stock up on Sexy Accessories

146

CHAPTER THIRTEEN

The Art of Talking Dirty

160

WEEK FOUR: MASTERING
YOUR MOJO!

170

CHAPTER FOURTEEN

Focus on Foreplay

171

CHAPTER FIFTEEN

Lingerie for Seduction

186

CHAPTER SIXTEEN

Exploring Fantasies

202

CHAPTER SEVENTEEN

Creating Flirtation

212

MOJO FOR LIFE!

221

CHAPTER EIGHTEEN

Taking Inventory

222

CHAPTER NINETEEN

*Even More Sexy Scenarios
for Now (or Later)*

228

CHAPTER TWENTY

Mojo Model Roundup

247

CHAPTER TWENTY-ONE

*You Did It! Now Keep
That Mojo Flowing!*

251

APPENDIX

261

ACKNOWLEDGMENTS

263

You, Me, and
the Mojo Makeover

H ELLO, GORGEOUS . . . WELCOME TO YOUR MOJO MAKEOVER!
I'm thrilled you've decided to take part in this fun,
fabulous, and deliciously foxy four-week journey to a sexier, more
confident, and more satisfied you. I'm going to be your guide for
the entire process, and seeing as we'll be spending the next thirty
days or so together, allow me to introduce myself . . .

As the cofounder of the sexy beauty and lifestyle brand Booty
Parlor, I've spent the last six years talking to women about sex. I
chat about it at work, the grocery store, yoga classes, cocktail
parties, and coffee shops; with girlfriends, A-list celebrities, and
strangers alike. I've led hundreds of private "Sexy Shopping
Parties," where I've shared Booty Parlor's products and philosophy
and inspired women to create sexier, more satisfying experiences
in their lives.

For as long as I can remember, I'd been the sexual sounding
board for friends and strangers, but there was a moment when the

lightbulb really went off—a moment when I realized that all of this talking about sex was actually the basis for a program that could transform women and their sex lives. My husband, Charlie, and I had just launched Booty Parlor and I was showcasing our products at a women's-only shopping event when I struck up a conversation with a woman there. I learned that she was single, and I cut right to the chase, asking her whether she was having orgasms by herself and whether she knew how to satisfy herself sexually. She looked at me like Bambi in the headlights—as in, *Mack Truck headlights*. As we continued to chat, I came to understand that she was in the dark about her own pleasure. No one had ever had that conversation with her, and no one—including herself—had ever given her permission to experience the incredible rush of happiness and release of a good old-fashioned orgasm. She'd made it well into her twenties without having had what I call a "sexy solo session." And since she didn't know how to reach orgasm herself, she'd never been able to climax with any of her boyfriends. She simply didn't have the tools or knowledge—but she had the enthusiasm to learn, and she was more than ready to start seeking out her own sexual satisfaction.

I explained how she could tune in to herself and turn herself on (which I'll soon share with you, too). Then I talked her through the basics of using the designer sex toy we'd selected for her. "Go slowly and let your body get used to the sensations," I said, "Even try it over your clothes at first. Close your eyes, remember to breathe, and just feel the rise—the new sensations that start to happen." Giving her further guidance, I said, "Start to move against the toy, find a rhythm, and try different levels of pressure and directions of motion. Mostly—explore! This is your orgasm. Take your own sweet time with it!" I answered some of her more detailed questions on reaching the Big O, and sent her off with a hug and a *You're going to love loving yourself!*

Yes, this is a pretty frank conversation to have upon first meeting someone, but this is my way. I believe every woman deserves the permission, knowledge, and tools to fully own her sexual satisfaction, so I just get straight to the point.

The next night, the same woman approached me again. This time she was literally running toward me from across the room—arms waving, smile beaming, aura simply *glowing*! "Oh . . . My . . . God," she said, "I can't believe what I was missing all this time!"

She exuded sexy self-confidence. She radiated energy. She was blissed out! It was as if she'd discovered a whole new, sparkling side of herself. She was turned on—to herself, to life. And all it took was a little girlfriend-to-girlfriend chat, a few simple instructions, and a new accessory to give her the inspiration she needed to create a mind-blowing, sexy experience. It became crystal clear:

A part of her had been *made over* through our interaction and her take-home experience. She had found a deeper, sexier, more confident relationship with herself. When a woman discovers this kind of inner sexiness and capacity for sexual satisfaction, she is a new woman. This is the power of a Mojo Makeover.

I decided that I wanted to help more women feel the way she did, and I started actively developing the concept of the Mojo Makeover. Since then, I've helped thousands of women create sexier lives that suit their unique personalities, preferences, and relationship statuses.

So, ask yourself, why are you here? You may be experiencing a setback in sexual desire or a dip in sexy self-confidence that are keeping you from feeling your foxiest. Maybe you want to lead a sexually confident, adventurous, and satisfying life, but you aren't sure where to start or how to make time for it. Or you may already have a strong sexy foundation and want to push your lusty exploration to the next level. No matter what you need, the Mojo Makeover can help you get there—and it works by building on *your* thoughts and feelings, *your* strengths and desires, and everything that makes you *you*.

ME, FROM MAKEUP TO MOJO

Back in high school, when I wasn't chasing rocker boys or caught up in after-school activities, I helped my mom at the beauty salon, where she was a successful makeup artist. My mom was always a total knockout: Foxy. Charismatic. Irresistibly cute. She somehow got out of every ticket a policeman ever tried to give her. She was a ballerina and an artist, and from her I learned a lot about embracing, exploring, and using my unique femininity and sex appeal.

But besides being gorgeous, my mom was an incredible makeup artist with the ability to transform women through her makeovers. She'd make sunshine pour out of women's eyes as they looked in the mirror, happily transfixed by their own revealed beauty. Sometimes she'd illuminate their inner sirens, and they'd look at themselves with an evening of seduction in mind. Other times, it was a simple makeup solution that showed the woman she was just as beautiful on the outside as she felt on the inside.

I noticed how quick women were to diminish themselves when they'd sit in her chair, immediately announcing how awful their noses were, how they wished they had higher cheekbones, and remarking on countless other perceived flaws.

But no matter how self-critical they were initially, they would all relax when Mom started asking them questions. She wanted to know about *their* lifestyles—were they stay-at-home moms? Traveling businesswomen? Did they like to host funky dinner parties or throw backyard barbecues? What were *they* looking for? Once she knew about their lives, she'd help them create workable and effective beauty regimens. If a harried working mother needed to apply her face in under five minutes, my mom created a quick and easy routine and taught her how to replicate it at home. She always played to her clients' strengths: their best natural features. She never tried making them over into someone they weren't, and her clients always left feeling happier.

Through watching my mother work over the years, I learned to believe in the beauty and power that exists in every woman. I came to understand that with a little girlfriend-to-girlfriend chat, some practical instruction, and yes, a little lip gloss, you could help any woman discover her unique beauty, feel more alive, and boost her inner confidence. So, starting Booty Parlor and becoming a Sexy Lifestyle Expert was a very natural evolution for me. Through my mother's business, I understood how makeup and beauty rituals help a woman look and feel beautiful, confident, and sexy. Through my own sexual experiences, I learned about the positive, confidence-boosting effects of personal pleasure and became my friends' go-to girl for sex advice. And in my professional career as the founder and Sexy Lifestyle Expert for Booty Parlor, I've educated thousands of women on sex and sexy products (both one-on-one and in groups). All of this has prepared me with the necessary knowledge and experience to create and lead you through this Mojo Makeover program.

One thing you can be sure of. The Mojo Makeover won't try to change you into something you're not. We're going to take what you've already got and enhance it, firing up your self-confidence and giving you the tools to create sexier experiences both inside and outside the bedroom. We're going to get you more in tune with your authentically sexy self!

YOUR MOJO MAKEOVER EXPERIENCE

I believe sex and sexiness are as important as eating, drinking, and working out, and yet more often than not, so many of us are willing to set sex aside, dismiss its importance, or simply let it drift to the back burner of our busy, multitasking daily lives. And that's where we get into trouble.

Focusing on your sexiness and making sex an integral part of your daily life might be new experiences, and maybe they're a path you've yet to navigate. You may even think they're selfish or frivolous. (They're not!) Thus far, you may have spent your life focusing on your intellectual development, building your professional career, reaching your peak level of fitness, defining your sense of fashion and style, becoming a great wife and mom, or finding charitable causes to dedicate your time to. And all that is fab! But listen up—while you should continue to do and value all these things, I need you to make some room to shine up your Mojo, too.

In fact, when you become the sexiest, most fabulous and vibrant version of you—with full-throttle confidence, self-love, and an active pursuit of the sexual satisfaction you deserve—all of your life's other endeavors will benefit. If you think you shine at the office, make the world's best wife, or have a personal style that's second to none, just wait until your Mojo is on fire!

But you'll still be yourself. The Mojo Makeover process isn't about changing who you are—it's about highlighting everything that you already are, drawing on your passions, your personality, your past experiences, and your current preferences and relationships. It's a formula for you to express the sexiest, most confident version of yourself. It's all about tapping into what's uniquely sexy about you. Think of it as your own personal sexual revolution. I've now done Mojo Makeovers with thousands of women across the country, and time after time I see incredible results. Imagine what a nation of Mojo-maxed women could accomplish. That revolution starts with you.

Make no mistake. The Mojo Makeover is a *lot* of fun, but it's also going to require hard work, honesty, and devotion to yourself (and your partner, if you so choose). You can't go from zero to multiorgasmic in sixty seconds. Part of the experience will be dedicated to healing old wounds and hang-ups so they stop hanging around. Instead, they'll become a part of your rich history and something you draw upon to determine what you do and don't want today.

As I walk you through the Mojo Makeover, I'll also share stories of my own journey to creating a sexy lifestyle. Like you, I've dealt with Mojo-zapping habits, bouts of low self-esteem and body confidence issues, hang-ups, bad choices, stress, and even depression. But through trial and error—and by creating and doing the exercises in this book—I learned how to cultivate my own wickedly vibrant sexy self-confidence and to create a smashing sex life with myself and with my husband. Yes, I said *with myself*! Along the way, I realized I could be my own best lover and my own best friend. We often forget that the relationship that lasts the longest—and as such, is the most important—is the one we have with ourselves. You might worry that this is selfish, but it's not. It's sexy self-care, and there's a big difference between the two.

Throughout our lives, our Mojo continues to change and evolve, contract and expand. It's my hope that you can always turn to the Mojo Makeover for help and inspiration, and a little tune-up when you need it. No matter where you are in life or what you're doing, you can never give up on your Mojo!

So are you ready to get your Mojo running? Let's get started!

THE OFFICIAL

booty parlor

MOJO

MAKEOVER

CHAPTER ONE

Introducing
the Mojo Makeover

R IGHT ABOUT NOW, YOU MIGHT BE EXCITED AND INTRIGUED,
curious and full of questions, or maybe even a little
intimidated. Don't worry; I'm going to ease you in to this process
slowly! Before we get started on our journey, I'm going to lay out
the Mojo Makeover program plan so you can see how it'll work to
awaken your inner vixen.

WHAT IS MOJO?

If we're going to be making *it* over, we should probably discuss
what *it* is! In basic terms, your Mojo isn't so much a physical thing
as it is a feeling. Think of it as your feminine sexual spark. It's that
glow that comes from within, your lust for life, love, and sex, and
all the juicy possibilities that live therein. It is, in essence, your
sex—your sexual attitude, your sexual drive, your personal sexual

magnetism, and a reflection of how free you feel to express yourself sexually. Mojo is more than just confidence—it's sexy self-confidence; your ability to know, embrace, and love your body; to know what turns you on and satisfies you, and to then be able to communicate it.

THE MOJO MAKEOVER ACTION PLAN:
AN OVERVIEW

The Mojo Makeover is a four-week sexy lifestyle makeover plan that's easy to follow, seriously freeing, feminine, and oh so satisfying! To some of you, four weeks might seem like a long time to focus on your sex life and inner Mojo. But Rome wasn't built in a day, and neither was Angelina Jolie's sexy swagger! This is a lifelong organic change that we're going after—and that requires real work and a real commitment to yourself. Dedicating yourself to thirty days of lovely, lusty personal work can do a lot to break the Mojo malfunctions you've been experiencing, and help you to form new healthier, sexier habits.

During your Mojo Makeover, you'll shed any fears or doubts about the innate sexiness that's inside of you. The process is gentle and fun, but at times daring, too. You'll be challenged to look inside for the real you, pull her out, and get her out there in the world. So what should you expect?

♥ **A kickoff questionnaire.** This will help you indentify your Mojo Model—which is your *current* sexy lifestyle persona. The results will reveal how you're feeling about your sex life right now and shed light on the issues that brought you to this makeover and the areas you want to improve upon. You'll identify your goals and make a pact with yourself to change, grow, and unleash the sparkling, fired-up, sexual creature that you truly are.

♥ **Weekly activities.** These are designed to help grow your Mojo. These will prompt you into action and start to unlock your inner sexual radiance. You'll write in a journal, restock your closet with sexier clothes, experience the pleasure of "you time," and even master some seductive stripper moves for good measure. And there's *plenty* more.

♥ **Real-world advice.** Along the way, you'll be encouraged by testimonials from real women just like you—the brave, beautiful souls who've completed their own Mojo Makeover journeys. Some of them are married, some single, and they represent a wide range of backgrounds, belief systems, and sexual orientations. Their stories, called Mojo Moments, will be spotlighted to boost you up and give you real inspiration and insight.

♥ **A maintenance plan.** When our four weeks together are complete, I won't leave you or your Mojo high and dry. With the Mojo Maintenance plan, you'll be fully equipped with all the tips, tricks, and tools you need to keep your sexy revolution going. And to wrap things up in a deliciously foxy bow, I'll share my tried-and-true Mojo Maintenance spell, which has worked for me and countless other women.

Through it all, I'll urge you to express yourself fully and truthfully, to take some leaps of faith, and to push yourself out of your comfort zone. I'm going to ask you to work through your hang-ups, letting go of bad habits and thought patterns that no longer serve you. It's likely that no one has ever asked you to think about sex this much, so it may feel strange at first, or even unnecessary. But trust me when I tell you it'll all be worth it!

THE TOOLS FOR YOUR MAKEOVER

Whether you're currently a vibrator aficionado or a total beginner, sex toys will play an important role in your Mojo Makeover. So let's leave the taboos and outdated stigma surrounding them behind us. It's simple: You can't get a makeover at a beauty counter without brushes, colors, and an eyelash curler. You can't transform your hairstyle without scissors. You can't make over your sex life without some tools, either!

But when I use the term *tools,* I'm referring to a wide range of provocative accessories that'll help inspire your sexy self-confidence and enhance the creation of new sexy experiences. That can mean lingerie and toys, props and potions, even sexy beauty products. And tools can be something you use on your own or share with your partner.

Despite what you might be thinking, you really don't need any previous knowledge or experience with bedroom accessories—just an open mind. A crucial component to a successful Mojo Makeover is your enthusiasm to try new things and not let anything—like preconceived notions or judgments—get in the way of your exploration, progress, and the *wow* experiences you're going to have!

SUPPLIES

YOU'LL NEED

❖

As we're getting ready to begin, you'll need to pull together
some simple supplies to set the stage for your makeover.

❤ **A journal.** It doesn't have to be pricey, just representative of your personal style so that you'll want to use it.

❤ **A stack of fashion and celebrity magazines.** If budget is a concern, ask your friends whether they have any extras.

❤ **A corkboard or large piece of construction paper.** You'll be using this to create your Mojo Motivation Board.

❤ **"School supplies."** Also for the board, pick up some pushpins, glue sticks, scissors, and other

inspirational tidbits—think sequins, feathers, strips of lace, whatever textures and fabrics make you feel sexy!

❤ **A full-length mirror.** You'll be spending a lot of time worshipping yourself in it over the next four weeks.

❤ **What else?** Along the way you'll have opportunities for a bit of shopping. Lingerie, sex toys, and other Mojo gear will accessorize your experience—but don't worry if you're not ready to pick those up quite yet. We'll get there!

HOW THE MOJO MAKEOVER
WILL WORK FOR YOU

I don't want to sound like I'm trying to sell you a line, but it's true: the Mojo Makeover works. I've seen it work equally on women who are single and coupled up, thin and voluptuous, shy and extroverted, young and old . . . and the common thread is that each woman was dedicated to the process. If you commit, it will work. The only women it hasn't worked for are those who never try it.

At the end of the four weeks, you'll emerge with a radiant glow, knowing yourself in a more intimate way. Your sexual horizons will be broader and far more gorgeous. You'll be more confident both in and out of the bedroom. You'll feel more passionate about yourself, which will in turn lead others to feel more passionately about you, too. Even strangers will take notice and want what you've got! You'll elicit double- and triple-takes. You'll inspire other women simply by being the sexiest, most confident version of yourself!

HOW MORE MOJO
HAS HELPED OTHER WOMEN

In addition to the personal Mojo Makeovers I've done, the program has been influenced by the stories and findings from my field of Sexy Lifestyle Advisors— the thousands of women across the country doing Booty Parlor Sexy Shopping Parties every night of the week. They're reaching a diverse cross-section of women with the Mojo Makeover experience in every part of the country and then sharing their real stories with me so that I can share them with you! The most common (if you want to call them common!) transformations we've all seen include:

- 💜 Massive increases in sexy self-confidence, self-love, and self-acceptance.
- 💜 Heightened enthusiasm for sex.
- 💜 Amplified confidence and knowledge to talk about sex.
- 💜 Intensified sexual satisfaction (both with and without partners).
- 💜 Huge improvements in the orgasm department—both in quantity and quality!

Check out two of my favorite Mojo Model moments from women who have been transformed by the Mojo Makeover!

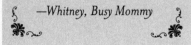

MOJO MOMENT

Diving into the Mojo Makeover was tough. I was so stuck in my daily routine with my toddlers that I completely forgot about my love life. But when I started going through the process, it became painfully obvious that a giant part of my marriage was being neglected and needed to be revived, not just for my husband but also for me! Sex is the fun part about marriage, so why do *so* many of us rank it so low on the to-do list! The Makeover made sex fun again!

—Whitney, Busy Mommy

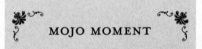

MOJO MOMENT

The Mojo Makeover not only spiced up my boyfriend's and my sex life, but also rebirthed that element of discovery and newness that often fades in longer-term relationships. Most important, it made me more acutely aware of my wants, needs, sexuality, and confidence—which translated not just into my relationship, but other areas of my life, as well.

—Suzette, Frustrated Fox

BEFORE YOU START ...

Now that you're clearer about your Mojo Makeover path, it may have raised some questions. Let's look at the ones I'm most frequently asked at the onset of a Mojo Makeover:

Do I include my partner?

Maybe you're married or otherwise coupled up and you have concerns about whether to include your partner in your makeover experience. I encourage you to do what you feel best suits your personal journey. If you think that your partner will enhance the experience, involve him. And if you feel that it's something you'd like to cherish on your own, that's okay, too! There's no right or wrong answer to this question—do what your instinct tells you to and you can never go wrong.

Will my menstrual cycle affect my makeover?

At some point during the Mojo Makeover, it's likely that you're going to get your period—and that can mean feeling randy one minute, then completely disinterested the next. But it doesn't have to derail your Mojo Makeover. The best cure for PMS moodiness is hot sex. Trust me, nothing resets your psyche like a mind-bending orgasm!

What if I'm a perfectionist?

It's easy to get flustered when you're learning something new. Don't get down on yourself! The Mojo Makeover is a process of self-discovery. There will be days when you'll feel like you're floating on a sparkling pink cloud of orgasmic delight and days when you'll feel full-on frustrated. Remember—being loving and kind to yourself is an important part of the process, and setbacks are just opportunities for growth. Just keep trying!

Can I turn to my friends for help?

Yes! You should seek out friends to share your experience, excitements, and concerns. Think of them as your personal cheerleaders who are on call to support you through this. You can reach out to the girls to keep you motivated, whether you've just tried an awesome new bedroom move and you want a pat on the back or you're frustrated and need a little pick-me-up.

How much of the process is work and how much is pleasure?

Learning new lifestyle skills may sometimes feel challenging, but this sexy transformation program should be juicy, spicy, decadent, frisky, and fun—and you need to remember that, especially in the tough moments. So if you fall while practicing your sexy walk in stilettos or feel ridiculous when trying out a new seduction scenario, have a good laugh! And if you need to cry it out, do that, too. Dedicate yourself wholeheartedly to the experience, and you'll reap the rewards—I promise.

DITCH ANY "I CAN'T" EXCUSES

Hard work is just that—hard. I know you're busy and you might be tempted at times to step away from this journey. When you feel excuses creeping up, flip back to this list. It'll help put you back on your path.

I'm too busy.

Aren't we all? These days, everyone has a busy multitasking life, and that's exactly why you should stick with the program. You're just as important as everything else you do in your life, if not more so! It's time to make time for you and your sex life.

I feel silly.

At first it can feel silly or strange to dance in front of your mirror in your underwear or find the courage to tell your lover what you truly desire. But silly is good! It means you're breaking out of your comfort zone and opening yourself up to new and delicious experiences. Plus, relaxing into the discomfort prepares you for the often ridiculous and unpredictable moments that naturally happen during sex.

Maybe sexy isn't what I'm supposed to be.

Though you may not be a believer just yet, I promise that there's a sexier, more satisfied version of you just waiting to come out and play. It's not about living up to some external standard of sexy; it's about discovering what's uniquely sexy about you and helping it shine brightly! You're meant to be and feel sexy. There's an inner vixen in there somewhere, and she's uniquely your own.

My partner thinks this is nonsense.

It can be difficult and annoying when you have an unsupportive partner who makes fun of the journey you've chosen. Just remember—this whole process is for *you*. And while your partner may benefit from the results, the ultimate goal is for *you* to realize *your* sexiest self. Stay focused on that. Typically, once your partner catches on to your sexy new groove, he'll quickly get onboard and start supporting your quest. And who knows what kind of arousing adventures that might lead you on?

All right, sweet thing, sharpen your pencil and get ready—next up, it's time for you to take the Mojo Makeover questionnaire!

CHAPTER TWO

The Mojo Makeover Questionnaire

IDENTIFYING WITH WHAT I LIKE TO CALL YOUR "MOJO MODEL" IS A way to gain understanding of yourself and those around you. It can also give you a sense of belonging and community because once you identify yourself as, say, a Busy Mommy, you'll be sure to find other Busy Mommies in your world who'll want to learn what you're learning! But know that your Mojo Model isn't just about defining yourself and bonding with other women. It will also help you see how your Mojo is malfunctioning, which in turn will help you map out your goals for the Mojo Makeover process.

WHERE THE MOJO MODELS COME FROM

Through my constant sex chatter with women at events and parties (and with my girlfriends, too), I began to notice common themes. My ears were flooded with stories of women's body insecurities. I was shocked to hear how little emphasis women were placing on their own sexual satisfaction, and how little time was being dedicated to having orgasms! Sex drives were low, hang-ups were high . . . but it wasn't all sexual doom and gloom.

I was also wowed by some amazingly turned-on women! There were women having lots of orgasms, and women with adventurous, communicative lovers in their lives. Some of the women I met were having lots of sexy solo sessions and were enthusiastic and open to exploring new sensual experiences. And then there were those who had tried it all and wanted to try even more!

After talking to hundreds and hundreds of women, I noticed definite patterns that were dictated by a woman's phase of life and that closely influenced her sexual self-perception. Some women were mommies, while some were newly engaged, married for ten years, or struggling to find a special long-term love. Some women were wild, adventurous, and sexually expressive by nature, and others really wanted to be but weren't sure how to cultivate that part of themselves. And so my advice started to take on a more tailored approach to address the needs of each woman's separate but common concerns. This is how the concept of the Mojo Model developed into what it is today.

You might be thinking, *Aren't there just two categories: women who aren't getting any and women who aren't getting enough—either in quantity or quality of sex?*

There's definitely some truth to this, but women are complex creatures, and associating with a more detailed Model will provide the opportunity for deeper, more specific insight and a richer makeover experience. There's so much more we're talking about than just having *sex*! We're developing confidence, inner light, self-love, acceptance, intimacy, forgiveness, and wild, unabashed bravery to discover our sexiest selves! Finding your Mojo Model will help you build all that more effectively, so let's go meet your Model.

THE QUESTIONNAIRE

RIGHT NOW, *I want you to focus on how you think about, feel, and experience your Mojo in this very moment—uninterrupted, without judgment, and with total honesty. Make sure you go through each Mojo Mind-set below, and score yourself based on how true each statement is to you. Use the scoring scale (right) to help guide your answers.*

SCORING SCALE

1 point—never
2 points—seldom
3 points—sometimes
4 points—often
5 points—always

Mojo Mind-set 1

3 1. I experience feelings of guilt about having sex and feel as though it's dirty. 4
2 2. I have trouble reaching orgasm and am sometimes unsure whether I've had one. 3
1 3. Faking orgasms is a part of my regular routine. 1
3 4. When I was growing up, sex education was about the birds and the bees, but little else. 5
2 5. I'm not honest with myself and my friends about sex. 3
TOTAL: 16   11   14

Mojo Mind-set 2

4 1. I've had an interest in sex from an early age. 2   2
1 2. I can be pretty demanding of my lovers. 1
1 3. I experiment, push boundaries, and explore my sexual life to the fullest. 1 1
4 4. Sex is an open topic of discussion for me. 3
1 5. My sexuality is a defining characteristic of my identity. 1   1
TOTAL: 8   11   8

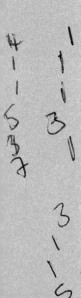

Mojo Mind-set 3

3 3
1. Sex comes only after everything else I have to get done in my day, if at all. (5 7

1 1
2. My kids are my top priority. (1

1 1
3. My sexual identity has changed since I had kids. | 5

4 4
4. I find it difficult to find the time to take care of and pamper myself. 4 5

3 3
5. My partner's drive is higher than mine. (5

TOTAL: 8   12   17   72   17

Mojo Mind-set 4

3 3
1. I feel my sex life lacks frequency and excitement. 3 5

3 4
2. I don't put as much effort into my sexuality now that I'm in a monogamous relationship. 2 6

1
3. It's easier for me to take care of my own orgasm rather than try to have one with my partner or instruct him on how to get me there. | 1

2 1
4. My and my partner's sex drives are often out of sync. | 5

1 3
5. More seductive experiences in my relationship would help me to feel desired. 3 3

TOTAL: 10   12   10   19   33

Mojo Mind-set 5

1 1
1. I've been single longer than I'd like. 3 1

3 4
2. I feel as if something is holding me back from going after the sex life, relationship, and intimacy that I desire. 4 5

3 3
3. I'm confident flirting but don't know how to close the deal. 5 5

5 5
4. I'm hungry to learn more about sex and my sexuality through an intimate relationship. 5 5

3 2
5. I'm mostly comfortable with my body but have anxiety over being naked with someone else. 25   15   19   3

TOTAL: 22   61   15

Now Find Your Mojo Model!

Tally up your score for each Mojo Mind-set and note the one you scored highest in (Mind-set 1, 2, 3, 4, or 5). Find the corresponding Mojo Model (they are numbered 1–5) on the next pages. That's your Model.

If you have two or more mind-sets with high or matching scores, go back through each high-scoring section and double-check your answers—are you really being 100 percent truthful with yourself? If your scores come out the same, read each definition that matches your high-scoring types and then pick the one that you most strongly connect with as your lead Mojo Model. It's very common for women to have overlapping Mojo Models, so simply keep both in mind as you continue on your Mojo Makeover. Each one can be equally as important to you in becoming the captivating sexual dynamo you want to be!

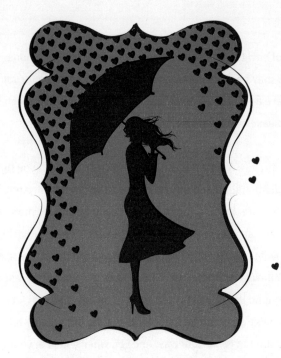

the pleasure virgin

THE BASICS. As the name suggests, you may have never had sex, but it's more
likely you're a "virgin" to real, authentic sexual satisfaction. Simply put,
you've got an inkling that there's more to sex—and more in it for you—but
you're a bit in the dark about how to figure it all out. You might've grown
up in a religious family where sex was a taboo subject and sex education
came in the form of the classic birds-and-bees chat (and maybe a peek at
some late-night Cinemax movies). Masturbation wasn't encouraged, so the

discovery of how to bring yourself to orgasm was limited to none. Intimacy with others may be more about going through the motions for you or doing it just to please a lover. In general, you don't feel confident enough in your moves to please both your lover and yourself.

WHAT TO LOOK OUT FOR. Years of unsatisfying sex may have left you tightly wound up in sexual frustration and unsure of how to unravel the mystery of your own personal pleasure, leading you to become complacent. It's more than likely you've become an expert at faking it. You're probably experiencing pleasure in some way, but you're either not allowing yourself the actual release or you don't know how to get there. You'll need to retrain your brain, especially if you carry around thoughts that sex and self-satisfaction are dirty. These thoughts act like an umbrella that blocks out the opportunity for experimentation to come your way. And yet, when you hear your girlfriends talk about sex, you often find yourself overcompensating by pretending you're in on the experiences they're dishing about when really you're not. That does a great disservice to you and your Mojo!

WHAT'S AHEAD. As you move through your Mojo Makeover, some of your main challenges are going to be overcoming sex guilt, letting go of your previous perceptions of sex, and learning how to honor your own feelings. You'll also need to slow down and spend some time with yourself to figure out your likes, dislikes, and what brings you to orgasm—and that means no more faking! Once you've figured that out, you're going to need to learn how to communicate it to your partner in a loving, constructive way.

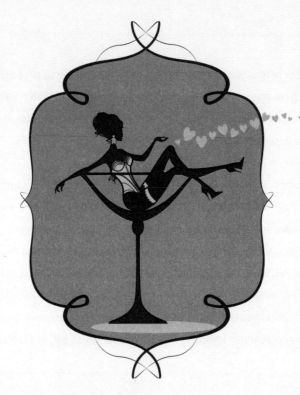

the adventure seeker

THE BASICS. You have good sex and relationships—which is what helps you be so
adventurous! But you tend to get stuck in ruts where it's all about the action
and less about the connection. Your *let's try anything* attitude and an
endless hunger for information are a great foundation upon which to explore
all aspects of your sexuality. When you were growing up, sex was likely a
more open topic in your household, which helped give you a healthy
self-esteem and openness about your body. You weren't afraid of society,

MODEL 2

family, or religious expectations about sex . . . and because of that, you didn't grow up with hang-ups. You consistently want to take your sexual explorations to even higher levels, but even you get stuck sometimes and may be unsure how to break through your plateau.

WHAT TO LOOK OUT FOR. Being caught up in adventure can be fun, but if you let yourself get too consumed by thrill seeking, you start to lose the intimacy and connection with yourself and your lover. If you get too demanding in the bedroom, it can frustrate your lover, and diminish his interest, leaving you unsatisfied. Sure, the experimentation is fun and frivolous, but can you ever just have "normal" intimate sex? And moving into a transitional phase—for example, changes that come with getting married or pregnant—can potentially create an identity crisis that could cause you to shut down or act out.

WHAT'S AHEAD. Your Mojo Makeover challenges will be to figure out how to find exciting new sexual experiences to keep you satisfied, while allowing yourself to make love and remember that it's okay to go back to the intimate basics. You're going to have to slow down a little to reconnect with yourself and find an identity beyond being a vixen or sex goddess. And you're going to discover new adventures in anticipation and letting go of control.

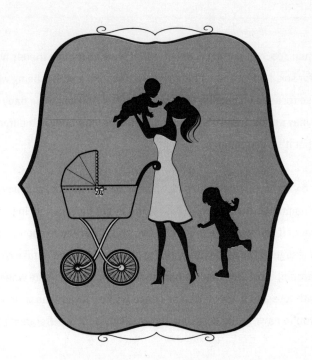

MODEL 3

the busy mommy

THE BASICS. Due to your hectic lifestyle—balancing family duties, career, and various outside influences—your attention to yourself and your sex life falls by the wayside, leaving you feeling frustrated and unsure of where your sexy, sassy self went! You often switch between many roles in your life, but because you're so expert at taking care of everyone else, you frequently forget to take care of yourself. At one point, you may have had an identity as a sexy social being, but when your child was born, you moved into the instinctual space of putting yourself last. It feels as though there's no time or space for sex, and it can be hard for you to feel like a sexual being when you're so focused on juggling your daily routine. And while the baby weight may or may not be gone, it's likely you're seeing your body in a different way after what it's been through.

WHAT TO LOOK OUT FOR. Whether it's because of time or money, you may not be getting pampered the way you used to. You might be experiencing some resentment if you're a stay-at-home mom, and when you're spending your days in charge of the homestead, you're often too drained to take charge in the bedroom, too. It can also be hard to feel sexy in your home when it's filled with toys and diapers. Your sex drive is likely lower than your partner's, and if you're having solo sessions, they're likely a lot less frequent than before.

WHAT'S AHEAD. Your number one Mojo Makeover issue? Making time for sex. But leading into that, you're going to have to desire yourself and find yourself desirable again! Even if you can take five minutes to do something that makes you feel good, it will make a world of difference. You'll need to relearn how to communicate with your partner about sex, and relearn what your sex life means to you. But most of all, you need to remember who you were pre-baby, and figure out how to incorporate that into who you are now.

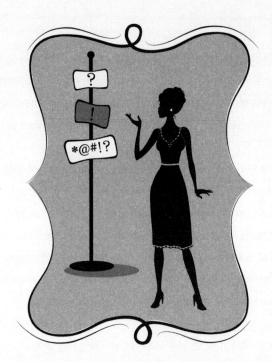

the frustrated fox

THE BASICS. Do you feel as if you're not having enough sex in your relationship or the sex you're having isn't satisfying enough? Welcome to your Mojo Model! Unfortunately, you feel a lot of unrest when it comes to your sex life. Sexual communication with your partner is breaking down, and you may be dealing with feelings of neglect (going both ways!). When you do have sex, you tend to just go through the motions. It wasn't always this way. Because you don't feel desired, you've stopped desiring your partner. You're bored with the routine and want to spice it up again, but you're not entirely sure how to make that happen. And on top of all that, you feel your relationship's sexual chemistry has faded, or you're finally noticing there was never chemistry to begin with. Whatever the reason, it's no longer feeding your sexual soul.

WHAT TO LOOK OUT FOR. If you're experiencing an imbalance of control in your relationship, it can contribute to making you feel unimportant. You might find solo sessions becoming your sexual activity of choice. You may feel you're always initiating the action, which doesn't make you feel wanted and eventually starts to slow your drive down even more. When you want to try to communicate about it, your partner may shut down. The result? Eventually, you wind up fantasizing about everyone but your partner.

WHAT'S AHEAD. During your Mojo Makeover, you're going to learn how to communicate with your lover, and if you can't, you're going to decide whether he's the right one for you. If there was once passion, you'll figure out how to bring it back by getting to the root of your sexual issues and breaking out of routines. But most of all, you'll be bringing sex back to your life, rediscovering yourself and your lover, and moving forward to a point in your relationship where sex becomes fresh and exciting again.

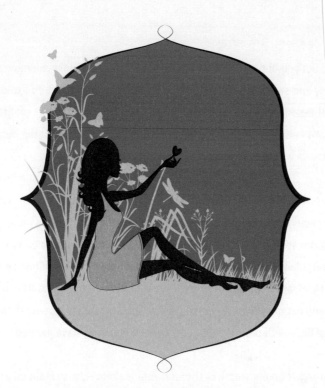

the late bloomer

THE BASICS. Picture a beautifully colored flower bud that's dying to stretch its petals to their full extent but unable to because it's not feeling enough of the heat from the sun. That's you! You've had some sex in the past, and some of it has been good, but you're single (and likely have been for some time), overall lacking confidence, and just can't seem to get your sex life going. Chances are, you're in a transitional phase, moving away from the woman you were into the woman you are, but now your dating and sex life need to catch up with you. You know how to work it and want to fully embody your inner vixen, but you don't know how to close the deal. And while you have a rich fantasy and solo life, you're stumped on how to parlay that into explosive sexual experiences with someone else! Chances are you didn't get attention from boys growing up, making you a bit of a late bloomer. But the best thing? You have a willingness to learn!

WHAT TO LOOK OUT FOR. While you're like a blank canvas looking to be slathered in gorgeous bright colors, sometimes you're intimidated at the prospect, which can send you backsliding into old habits. You can get a bit too comfortable with yourself, cocooning in your home instead of having a sexy social life—and that means there's a lack of flirting action. Shutting down happens out of self-preservation habits, and sometimes, you hold on to past connections with partners long after their shelf dates have expired.

WHAT'S AHEAD. Working your way through your makeover, your main focus will be to own and use your sexy power—and that's going to mean breaking out of your shell. You're going to have to learn how to truly fall in love with your body and yourself, and own every part of your history without letting it consume you. But by the same token, you're going to have to let go of those awkward or unsexy images of yourself from your past. And you will not only need to flirt, but you'll also need to know what to do with the attention once you get it—and you will!

Now that you know your Mojo Model, it's time to commit. Think of the creed that follows as you own call to arms.

THE MOJO MANIFESTO

Every Mojo Makeover I do starts with the Mojo Manifesto. It always helps the woman I'm working with make a firm commitment to the experience she's about to have, while reminding her of the key components of what a self-confident sexy lifestyle is all about.

So as we draw this chapter to a close and look toward rolling up our sleeves to getting into the real nitty-gritty, I invite you to read the Mojo Manifesto out loud and embrace its message of delightful discovery, lusty abandon, and fearless self-awareness!

IN PARTICIPATING IN MY MOJO MAKEOVER, I REJECT

- My tendency toward negative body banter and all the other Mojo-zapping behavior it encourages, like putting myself down, shying away from my unique sexiness, not finding confidence in myself, and comparing myself to other women.
- Denying myself pleasure and satisfaction in all aspects of a fabulously sexy lifestyle, engaging in poor sexual communication, and settling for a sex life that isn't 100 percent reflective of what I deserve.
- Anything that doesn't support, embrace, welcome, encourage, or guide me toward discovering and owning my sexiest self.

I BELIEVE IN

- Creating a personal sexy revolution that encourages knowing, loving, and embracing every aspect of my sexiest self with passion and gives me the confidence and courage to share it with others.

💜 The importance that sex plays in my life and how it can help me shine in every area of my life, and that every woman deserves to feel sexy, desirable, and satisfied.

💜 The sisterhood . . . and that I have a duty to help other women understand that our inner light is what leads us to deserving more, exploring more, and creating more sexy experiences that lead to seriously satisfying lives!

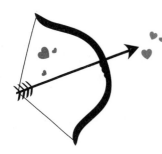

EXERCISE

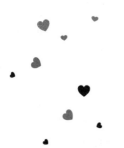

The "Before" Photo Session

Every good makeover includes a record of what the person looked like before and after the entire process, and the Mojo Makeover is no different. I want you to feel the difference within yourself and see it on the outside, too. The self-portraits you take today will be repeated in four weeks, after your work is complete, and their true value will become apparent then. Paste them in your journal for safekeeping.

So grab your camera. I want you to have a true image of who you are in your day-to-day as you are today. This will be your inspiration for your starting point.

💜 PHOTO 1 Running a daily errand

Take a picture of yourself dressed as you normally do when you go out in public for weekend errands (the grocery store, the mani-pedi place, watching a soccer game).

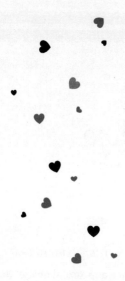

♥ PHOTO 2 Prepped for a night out

Catch an image of yourself dressed up to go out on the town. Whether it's out to a bar to meet your BFFs, a date with a new hottie, or a date night with your long-time love, snap away!

♥ PHOTO 3 You at your sexiest

Take a risqué picture, as racy as you feel confident with. Clothing is fine, but barer is even better. Stay in your comfort zone—it's okay!

♥ PHOTO 4 Post-orgasm

Take a portrait of yourself after you've had a great big orgasm. Take it while you're still in bed if you dare.

Whew! You've done a lot of work already, which is fantastic. You've found the Mojo Model you most closely identify with, you've had a chance to peer into your patterns and problems, and you might've even had some *a-ha* moments on what you'd like to accomplish through your makeover.

CHAPTER THREE

What Hinders Your Mojo

W**HAT EXACTLY IS A MOJO MALFUNCTION? IT'S ANYTHING THAT** gets in the way of your self-confidence and sexual desire. No matter what your Mojo Model, there are a few common obstacles experienced by most women on the path to fulfilling their sexiest potential. These Mojo-zapping monsters whittle away at your self-confidence and slowly drain your desire for sex—they suck the very life out of your ability to be fearless, foxy, and free. The longer you keep these behaviors around, the more they drain your Mojo and hold you back from being the amazingly alluring creature you're meant to be!

THE MOST COMMON MOJO MALFUNCTIONS

Before we start whipping your Mojo into shape, let's expose some stumbling blocks. Consider these wake-up calls, and then keep them in mind as you move through the chapters. The solutions will definitely be apparent over the next four weeks.

1. Negative body banter

One of the biggest Mojo zappers that I see time and time again is what I call negative body banter, which viciously gnaws away at our self-confidence. It's the self-destructive mental chatter we inflict upon ourselves, when we're down on our bodies and our beauty or when we compare ourselves negatively to other women. It can stem from having impossible, unrealistic goals for our physical selves. Somewhere along the way, we learned the message that our self-worth and self-confidence were directly linked to our size and external beauty.

This may have led to feelings of shame—shame that we're not thin enough or pretty enough, that we can't control our eating, our bodies, or our size. When you feel shame, you're not experiencing pleasure, because you feel you don't deserve it.

On the flip side, *positive* body banter or self-love—which you're going to learn a *lot* about in this book—shifts your focus to what your Mojo is really about: happiness, sexiness, freedom, and satisfaction—all of which you deserve. And you *will* get there, I promise!

2. Viewing sex as a chore

This malfunction is most common in women in long-term relationships. There was probably a time when you couldn't wait to get frisky with your lover, when the sex was spontaneous, the desire was high, and you sought it out with gusto. Now things are different. You're having sex once a week at best, and secretly, you could give *that* up; it's just not something you seem to need now. But you find yourself doing it to make your partner happy or to prevent your lover from being upset because you're not initiating it.

Yes, sometimes it's challenging to keep the desire alive—for yourself or your lover—and sometimes your to-do list is toppling you over and you're truly too tired. But remember how it used to be—at one point in your life you couldn't wait to have sex! You probably couldn't get enough. Sex is awesome. I'm going to help you remember that.

3. *Living a routine*

Do you find yourself doing the same thing over and over again in your bedroom routine, to the point where you can pinpoint when certain things will happen? It's time to break the cycle! Limiting your sexual experiences to what you've always known and what's always been comfortable means you're always going to get the same results. And that's . . . boring. Even if you're reaching orgasm, it can't be inspiring desire.

Personally, I see sex as a playground. It's a wonderful place to try new things and experience both my husband and myself in ever-changing ways. Sometimes that means having intimate, loving sex one day, and exotic, hungry sex the next. It also means having an open mind to explore new positions, roles, and environments that deliver pleasure. If I was doing the same thing every time, I'd miss out on all that creativity, raw expression, and emotional comfort—all of which consistently lead me to major awakenings, both physically and emotionally. And doesn't that sound delicious?

4. Not acting on frisky feelings

When I say *feeling frisky*, I'm referring to what starts as a little tingle in your brain or your lady parts that makes you think: sex! Frisky feelings have varying degrees of intensity, from a passing thought to must-have-it-now hunger. But frisky feelings don't mean a thing if you ignore them!

You might notice them when you're watching a hot scene in a movie or you catch a glimpse of your beloved looking particularly yummy as he emerges from a steamy hot shower. There's visual stimulation everywhere! The cute trainer at the gym (or his big barbell!), the silky sweetness of a chocolate-covered treat. And who hasn't had a morning where you awake from a dream where Robert Pattinson or Brad Pitt or Johnny Depp was very, very naked and there to please only you? If you push those randy feelings out of your mind and go about your day as if they never happened, you're missing out on a chance to boost your Mojo. I mean, if you're hungry, you eat, right?

When you wake up in the middle of that sexy dream, don't go back to sleep. Instead, grab your toy or your boy and cut loose! The more you pay attention to naughty moments—and act on them—the more sexual, and better, you'll feel.

5. Worn-down wardrobe

Wardrobe plays a special role in our lives as women. Cloaking yourself in ill-fitting jeans, faded undies, or curve-concealing tops is doing nothing for your sexy self-confidence. What you wear helps fuel and expresses your Mojo, giving you the daily opportunity to show off your sexiness and self-confidence everywhere you go (even if it's just to the laundry room).

Certainly your outer garments project a certain image to others, but it's really the body-touching pieces beneath those clothes that can set your Mojo on fire. News flash, ladies: you don't wear lingerie just for your lover; you wear it for yourself, to inspire your femininity, to accent your curves, pump up the girls, show off your gams, firm and smooth your bits, and actually to turn yourself on! Paying attention to—and having fun with—lingerie can do wonders for your sex life. The very act of paying attention to something so feminine inspires you to feel friskier and sexier.

Now I'm not saying you have to completely give up your favorite sweatpants, but when you look at your sweats, can you honestly say that they make you feel sexy? Probably not. I firmly believe that sexy can be comfy and comfy can be very sexy. And I'm going to show you how to pull it off for yourself. Having a wardrobe that makes you feel good and properly suits your body means instant Mojo!

6. Skipping basic sexy self-care

Pampering is a basic need for every woman. It can help you fire up your femininity and offers you the opportunity to connect to yourself. When you deny yourself self-care indulgences, you're neglecting yourself, and that diminishes your sex drive, leaving you to feel like a less-than-sparkling version of yourself. And who wants that? After all, silver has to be polished. Shouldn't you be doing the same thing for yourself?

You might think that spending time on sexy self-care is vain or a waste of time, but it's not. It's a feminine luxury that's essential to strengthening and maintaining your Mojo! This is about manicures, pedicures, bubble baths, and makeup—and it's also about eating well, sleeping well, taking relaxing baths, working out, and just taking time for yourself. Yes, it can be hard to do with the hectic lifestyles we all lead, but you need to boost your own Mojo with loving self-care if you want others to bask in its glorious glow. Trust me; once you start giving yourself five minutes here or ten minutes there, you'll see, and feel, a change for the better.

7. Poor sex-communication skills

No one can expect her lover to be a mind reader, as much as she'd like him to be! So if you're not talking about sex, your lover can't know what you need, what you're interested in, and what turns you on—or off. Staying silent—or worse, talking only on a surface level—depletes your Mojo and keeps you (and your partner) from finding your sexiest satisfaction. You may feel terrified to broach the subject at all, or you may just need some choice words to deliver your message in a kind, constructive way.

Whatever the reason, if you can't express your needs, they simply can't be met. Sex communication is as crucial as any other relationship communication— finances, children, family, and every other key point of discussion. Most important, you have to be willing to talk about all of it—the good, the bad, the everything in between. It's the only way to create the sex life you truly want and deserve. We'll dig into this thoroughly in an upcoming chapter, complete with scripts to help you find the words you need to get, and give, what you desire.

8. Holding on to sex guilt

It's not uncommon for women to have a dark part of their sexual history that left them feeling dirty or guilty or loaded them up with baggage that lingers around for years and years. You might have guilt from a religious upbringing, guilt from how your family dealt with sex, and even societal guilt about pleasure. But for you to become a fully realized sexual dynamo, you're going to have to let your guilt go.

If your sex guilt comes from a traumatic experience, you may feel that it was your fault that you put yourself in the position that led to those disturbing moments. But look at the situation again—you probably didn't know it was going to go the way it did. We often blame our former selves for situations that we didn't know how to prevent at the time because we were too young, too naïve, or too trusting.

What's most important is that you learn to forgive yourself and move forward. Building your sexy self-confidence is so crucial (and doable—don't worry!). In the weeks ahead, you'll find that you're denying yourself less often and, in turn, giving yourself permission to embrace and enjoy a new Mojo-rich path.

MOJO MEMO:

Letting Go of My Own Sex Guilt

Trust me when I say sexy self-confidence has not always come easy to me. I've gone through my growing and learning periods, too . . . and they weren't always graceful experiences. As a teenager, I was a star member of the *too much, too soon* club, where my enthusiastic pursuit of sexual experience occasionally left me feeling used, confused, and just plain terrible about my choices. I got myself into sexual situations that were out of my league, and thought that in order to grow into a woman, my sex appeal had to go into overdrive. I sometimes acted against my intuition, which always led to trouble and a nagging guilty inner voice that would ask, *Why'd you do that, Dana?*

After one exceptionally terrible choice I made, my mom put me in the car and dropped me off at a therapist's office. My parents had been open to discussing sex with me, but at that moment, they knew that I needed to talk to someone more equipped to listen to stories of my sexual missteps. This therapist allowed me to be remarkably honest—about what I'd been up to and how I was really feeling about it. It was so freeing! She helped me understand that my sexuality and desire could be a healthy, positive part of my life, where I made smart, safe choices that were in line with my intuition. She acknowledged that my desire for experience and adventure was normal—and that I shouldn't hold on to any shame for the mistakes I'd made.

The time I spent with her allowed me to deal with my feelings, move forward, and learn what was acceptable and healthy for me. She helped me "clean out my sexual closet," (which you'll be doing during Week One of the program). From there forward, almost all my sexual experiences were positive, exciting, expansive ones, and when they weren't, I was far more equipped to deal with them and move on. And that's what this week will be about for you.

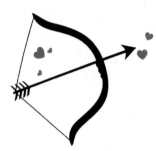

EXERCISE

Make a Mojo Motivation *Board!*

Now that you're aware of what's squelching your inner spark, it's time to start getting you fired up. This project will take time but it isn't hard. It's actually very cathartic. You're going to create a Mojo Motivation Board, a vision board that visually represents the sexiest "version" of you and the sexiest lifestyle you'd like to create.

The process of making a Mojo Motivation Board is thought provoking and fun, especially if you invite a girl-friend and do them together over cocktails! It'll focus your energy on the sexy universe you want to create, which is why this exercise is a key component to the Mojo Makeover. But it doesn't end with the creation of your board. You'll want to put it where you can see it every day, so that it acts as a regular reminder of what you're working toward. That in and of itself will help fire up your Mojo for the day!

How to create your personal board

Remember all those "school supplies" (like the cork-board, glue stick, and ribbons)? It's time to pull them out—along with that stack of magazines—and set aside an uninterrupted afternoon to channel your vision.

STEP 1: Set a creative, sexy mood by lighting some candles and turning on some inspiring tunes. Create an atmosphere that'll help get your Mojo moving in the right direction!

STEP 2: Go through your pile of magazines and clip images that are in line with the sexy lifestyle you wish to have. These could be images of celebrities or models whose style or sexy swagger you admire, sensual foods that make your mouth water, couples entwined in stolen lusty moments, dream bedrooms from architectural magazines that make you swoon, or words that inspire you to make sexier choices.

STEP 3: Don't limit yourself to just magazines. Consider collecting pieces of fabric that inspire the sexiness in you, like bits of lace that represent the lingerie collection you'd like to have. You can also put up buttons that help remind you of a fantasy where your beloved pops each of your buttons as he undresses you, rich and shimmering satin to remind you of what it would be like to get busy on sheets made of the same fabric, or maybe a patch of faux fur if one of your fantasies is to get frisky on a bearskin rug in front of a roaring fireplace . . . the possibilities are endless!

STEP 4: Start tacking down your goodies on the corkboard in a way that's totally your style, be it spare and orderly or a smorgasbord of elements that overlaps and flows over the board's edges.

STEP 5: Now it's time to find a home for your masterpiece! Ideally you should place it somewhere where you can easily and frequently see it, like on the wall of your closet. What's important is that it's somewhere where it can inspire you on a daily basis.

STEP 6: Bask in the sexy inspiration of your Mojo Motivation Board as much as you can, and drink in the sights of all the sensual indulgences you're going to infuse your life with!

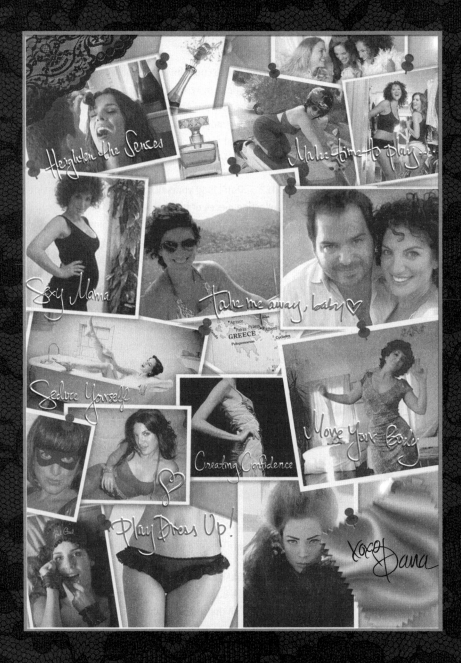

Heighten the Senses

Make time to play...

Sexy Mama

Take me away, baby ♡

Seduce Yourself

Creating Confidence

Move Your Body

Play Dress Up!

xoxo Dana

HERE'S MY PERSONAL
MOJO MOTIVATION BOARD!

Remember how I told you that these exercises were the result of tried and tested experiences that I've been through myself? Here's proof. To help give you inspiration, I wanted to share an image of my own Mojo Motivation Board and point out some of my favorite things on it.

Some of the things you'll notice on my Mojo Motivation Board are . . .

Playing dress-up

I have a thing for costumes, and Wonder Woman is my all-time favorite! Costumes are playful and sexy and always set me free.

Take me away, baby

Mmmm . . . this picture of Charlie and me is from a two-week vacation in Greece. We were so relaxed! And the fourteen-day sex marathon wasn't half-bad, either.

Sexy mama

This is a picture of me almost five months pregnant and still feeling über-sexy in one of my favorite stretchy tank dresses!

Heighten the senses

Indulging in the senses is super sexy to me. Chocolate, fruits, champagne, expensive perfumes. I'm a glutton for sensory stimulation!

Now that you've done a little introspection, I bet you have some thoughts about what you'd like to change in your sex life—things you want to stop doing, things you'd like to start (or start again). And that's exactly where I want you to be right now. You've got a base point to work from. Feel good about that because even though there's hard work ahead, it's all uphill from here!

MORE

BOARD BOOSTERS!

💗 **Put pictures of yourself on your board.** Choose shots where you feel you look your sexiest best or self-portraits where you were deeply, confidently connecting with the camera. What better way to send the message to the universe that this is the world you're looking to create for yourself?

💗 **Decorate your Mojo Motivation Board in ways that are uniquely you.** If you love sparkles, try some glitter glue around the frame of the corkboard to brighten it up; place stick-on gems on the pictures you love the most; put stars and hearts on others; play with paints. Lay quotes over photos. Or buy sheets of pretty wrapping paper and use it as a background.

💗 **Use affirmations.** You know, little one- or two-sentence pep-talk phrases. I want you to be especially on the lookout for phrases that give you permission to have what you deserve in your mental, emotional, and sexual life. You'll find plenty of examples in upcoming chapters.

💗 **Update it as you grow.** As your Mojo continues to fire up, you might find some things on your board aren't necessarily representative of you or your sexiest vision anymore . . . or maybe you've achieved the goal that a particular image represented. No worries—you can remove it, put a delicious new image in its place, and keep aiming higher!

This Week's Mojo Mission

CLEAN OUT YOUR SEXUAL CLOSET

I'm going to help you clear some mental space so you can start to create a more enthusiastic, satisfied sexy lifestyle. You'll sift through your past and present sexual experiences—the good and the bad—and in the process uncover the habits and hang-ups that cloud your Mojo. And from there, the real work begins.

GET READY TO

- ❤ Reprogram your wardrobe so every choice is a sexy, happy one.

- ❤ Uncover your Mojo malfunctions—the passion-robbing habits you might not even be aware of.

- ❤ Adopt new self-loving rituals that will make you feel more confident from head to toe.

CHAPTER FOUR

Give Your Wardrobe a Mojo Makeover

I KNOW YOU'VE PROBABLY HEARD THIS BEFORE, BUT YOU FEEL THE way you look, right? When you're consistently throwing on sloppy clothes, you start to feel sloppy. When you hide your body under ill-fitting pieces, you start to shrink away in social situations. Your wardrobe is the outer representation of your inner self and, of course, your Mojo. So, when your wardrobe is working, when your clothes are accenting your best assets, it's a major mood lifter and you're ready to shine—and that means insta-Mojo.

There are some great books on how to do a full fashion makeover, but for now, let's give your wardrobe its own minimakeover, shaking out the cobwebs and shaking up your Mojo! Adding a little sex appeal to your wardrobe will help you to look at yourself in a different way. Whether you're a Busy Mommy or a Late Bloomer, foxing up your wardrobe will help make that ultimate sexy vision of yourself more realistic. You'll want to carve out at least three hours for this, so grab some emergency snacks to keep you energized . . . and start digging!

STAGE 1:
PREP WORK

Make some notes on what your fashion hallmarks used to be, then read them through and decide which ones stand out to you as still being a part of you today.

- ♥ **Start to define what's sexy for you right now.** Is it gorgeous flowing shapes, classic wrap dresses, sumptuous fabrics, and jewel-tone colors? Reference your Mojo Motivation Board for inspiration. Then make a list of what you love.

- ♥ **Lose your attachment to what was sexy for you five, ten, twenty years ago.** That doesn't mean you can't carry hints of it through your life, but if we stay stagnant, how can we evolve?

- ♥ **Allow yourself to mentally catch up.** You'll want to create a new sexy style that reflects who you are *right now* in life. For example, maybe cleavage used to be your calling card in your twenties, but perhaps now it's your collarbone or nape.

STAGE 2:
DIGGING THROUGH

Get three garbage bags. One will be for alterations, another for donations, and the last for garbage.

- ♥ **Start sorting through your drawers and closets, evaluating each item.** Try things on to make sure they fit. If an article's not worth

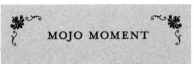

MOJO MOMENT

When my twins were tiny, just being showered was a big deal for me because they needed my attention all the time. But then time passed and I stayed in that mind-set. It's one of those things you don't realize is bringing your Mojo down until you stop. Well-fitting jeans and a few cute tops made me feel a million times better. I've also swapped unisex sweats for hip-hugging yoga pants. Small change, big gain!

—*Julia, Busy Mommy*

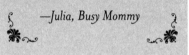

altering or you haven't worn it in a year, toss it into the donations or garbage bag. Things to toss? Schlubby workout wear, bras with fraying elastic, socks with holes in the toes, and any underwear you would be terrified to be caught in by a new lover (whether you're looking for a new lover or not!).

💜 **Pay attention to details.** What do you see that sparks you up and makes you feel immediately sexier? Is it a lace trim? Sequins that draw the eye to your sexy bust? Buttons that might inspire . . . unbuttoning? A particular shape that cinches your waist and highlights your hourglass proportions? Make note of these details; even if you decide not to keep those items, something about them has inspired you and you're one step closer to defining a sexier style.

💜 **Keep only what fits, what feels fresh, and what looks cute, today.** I know it's tempting to save the items you think you'll fit into one day. But how long have they been in your closet? Start honoring your sexy bod today with clothes that fit and flatter.

STAGE 3:
RESTOCK

Quickly schedule a day to visit the tailor for alterations and a visit to Goodwill. Do *not* go dipping back into those trash bags!

💜 **Review what's left in your wardrobe, and how you can make it work for you.** Surf style sites and thumb through fashion magazines for looks that you think are sexy and, most important, that you connect with as being sexy for you *right now*.

💜 **You should also have a sense now of what you need.** Do you have some great-fitting jeans, but you find yourself without sexy, sophisticated dresses for dinner dates? Did you find some fabulously flattering tops and tees, but come up empty-handed in the lingerie department? Make a wish list of items you want and need to sex up your closet now that it has all this extra room.

💜 **Grab the girlfriend you think has the best sense of style and hit the stores to explore the sexy new looks you've got your eye on.** Don't be afraid of the dressing room or not being 100 percent sure how to pull it together! Just try, try, try. Don't worry about buying; just start exploring what feels sexy on you.

💜 **Look for moments in your day that give you the opportunity to boost your Mojo by dressing a little sexier.** For example, slide on a lacy slip between your shower and dressing, and you'll feel far flirtier as you sip coffee and apply your makeup than you would in just your towel. Slither into something seductively soft after work but before bed. On Sundays, wear something that's both sexy and comfy while doing laundry. Trust me—puttering around the house in cuddly but suggestive clothes (instead of your trusty college-era sweats) will help you create a sense of everyday hotness!

REPLENISHING YOUR WARDROBE

You've cleaned, tossed, donated, and pulled together a few basics that make you feel sexy. I hope you've thrown out all your worn underwear! Now, set aside some money to treat your wardrobe (and your Mojo) to a few sexier items. When you're shopping, focus on accenting a physical feature you find sexy, no matter what that might be—your bust, bum, shoulders, collarbone, or even your eyes. Don't forget about colors that inspire you and the feel of the fabric against your skin. If it's scratchy and making you itch like crazy, it's guaranteed you're not going to be feeling sexy in it!

Mojo-friendly basics every wardrobe should have

💜 **Sweaters.** Boys love girls in tight sweaters. They're soft, textural, and curve hugging, and can show off your best above-the-waist assets.

💜 **Camisoles.** They can be worn as outerwear at work with a professional skirt and cardigan. You can easily transition into evening, making the look more seductive by adding a stiletto and taking off the cardigan, showing off your smooth, sexy shoulders.

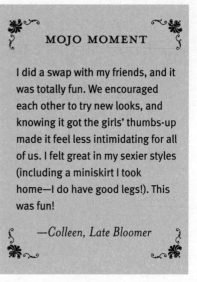

MOJO MOMENT

I did a swap with my friends, and it was totally fun. We encouraged each other to try new looks, and knowing it got the girls' thumbs-up made it feel less intimidating for all of us. I felt great in my sexier styles (including a miniskirt I took home—I do have good legs!). This was fun!

—*Colleen, Late Bloomer*

💜 **Button-down shirts.** Though they seem like they're a boring fashion fixture, they're easy to sex up! Put a button-down shirt on over a lacy cami and leave the buttons undone (or tie it at your rib cage, Daisy Duke style), and suddenly, you have a sexy wardrobe staple.

💜 **A little black dress.** A timeless sexy basic that can be dressed up or down. You can layer it with tights, boots, a sweater, or a shrug for a more casual look or dress it up with great accessories and heels.

If a wardrobe-replenishing trip to the shops isn't in the cards for you right now, it just means you have to be a little more creative! Organize a fashion swap with friends, encouraging everyone to bring the sexier items from their wardrobe that they're ready to part with. Donate what's left over to a good cause.

I stand by my belief that confidence is the sexiest thing a woman can have, and of course, you have to be comfortable to feel confident. Get your wardrobe humming in its sultriest, sassiest way, and you can be all three: comfortable, confident, and sexy!

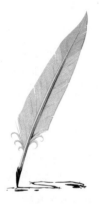

**JOURNALING
EXERCISE**

Ready to See a Shift in Your Self-confidence?

Grab your journal again, and make a list of sexy compliments you'd love to receive when you sport your new sultry sense of style. Want someone to tell you they love your gorgeous legs (now that people can see them, since you're wearing skirts more), or that your chic new jeans make your butt look amazing? Write it down, then post the list next to your bathroom mirror and choose a new one to tell yourself every day! Compliments, even—and especially!—from yourself, help you feel fabulous. And the more fabulous you feel, the more compliments you're going to get from people who notice you!

You've done some letting go, figuratively and literally. It feels good, right? You feel less weighed down, and hopefully, that *space* is primed and ready to be filled with sexy energy. Good work!

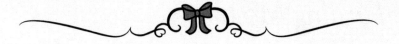

DON'T PUT THE JOURNAL AWAY JUST YET.
YOU'LL BE USING IT A LOT IN THE NEXT CHAPTER,
TO HELP UNDERSTAND YOUR DESIRES AND PERMIT
YOURSELF TO EMBRACE THEM.

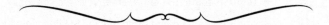

CHAPTER FIVE

Turning Mojo Malfunctions into Mojo Musts

N OW IT'S TIME TO REALLY SOLIDIFY YOUR MOJO MISSION through some thoughtful creative exercises that will help you push through some major Mojo blocks. Staying vigilant against these malfunctions is something to start early on in the process. Start practicing these tricks now, and by the end of the four weeks, they should be second nature!

1. GET A QUICK MOOD ADJUSTMENT

I want you to always feel as foxy and fabulous as you possibly can, but let's face it—we're all going to have bad days, when we'd rather curl up with a vat of pasta and a brick of chocolate. I call it the Funk—when what should be a short-term bad mood turns into a gloomy Funk that lingers for hours or sometimes days or weeks. Though bad moods are a perfectly normal part of life, leaving those feelings unresolved for too long can depress your Mojo, which can turn you off from you—from feeling alive and able to express your sexiness in everyday life. Sometimes the simplest things can send you spiraling downward, ruining your chances for a sexy experience!

For example, let's say you had a romantic date planned with your honey, and you were slated to meet up with him right after work. You spent all day thinking about how hot the postdinner sex would be, until you had a run-in with a psycho coworker at the office. You lost your temper; you can't calm yourself down again; the incident replays in your head over and over like a broken record; and before you know it, all those racy pre-date feelings have disappeared! That's why I want to give you these easy fixes to help you get out of a bad mood before it works its way into you too deeply and before it derails your Mojo.

So next time you find yourself in one of the following situations, try this exercise: see whether one of these love-yourself quick fixes doesn't help you out of it a little faster, restoring the bounce in your step and putting the sparkle back in your eyes.

SELF-CONFIDENCE SINKER	♥ YOURSELF MOVE
Feeling blue or just generally down . . .	Perk yourself up! Listen to happy music, watch a movie you love, or call a girlfriend for support and laughter. Make yourself smile, even if it feels forced. Watch your mood brighten instantly!

SELF-CONFIDENCE SINKER	♥ YOURSELF MOVE
Mooning over a fight you had with your lover . . .	Get out of the house. Go for a walk or hike, and let those endorphins take over. They'll help you clear your head for better communication when you return, too.
Letting your boss make you feel underappreciated . . .	Appreciate yourself! Write yourself work-related affirmations on Post-its and stick them around your workstation, telling yourself what a good job you do. Don't go bitching to coworkers—spewing negativity never helps in the long run.
Allowing a misunderstanding with your friend to ruin your day . . .	Understand yourself. Reminding yourself of all the things that make you a wonderful friend will help you feel better while you allow your friendship some breathing room. Then, hug it out.
Being so wrapped up in stress that you can barely breathe . . .	Step away, if even for a moment. Get a good salt or sugar scrub and slough those stress gremlins away, then sink into a luxurious bubble bath to help you melt into bliss. If you don't feel that you have time for a bath, even a quick hot shower followed by a fresh towel can do wonders for your outlook.

2. STOP COMPARING YOURSELF
TO OTHER WOMEN

It's such a tempting trap to fall into, isn't it? You're walking down the street, feeling super confident and irresistible, and then you spot . . . *her*. You know, she of the luxuriously shiny hair, legs that seem to go on forever, and an air that suggests she's not only got *it*, she *knows* she's got it—and what's more, she doesn't seem to care that men are falling over themselves to get to her! Suddenly all those self-assured, positive, bold feelings you were having whoosh out of you and you're instantly contemplating and comparing how your differences set you apart.

I had this Mojo malfunction, big time. After college, I was a cocktail waitress at a very hip nightclub in New York City. All around me were these model-like beauties—my fellow waitresses were hot! If they weren't tall and skinny, then they looked exotic, with almond-shaped eyes and sexy, flowing hair. There I was, the frizz-prone redhead, with a curvy bod and average height. As with most clubs, if the customers liked your look, they tipped better, so there was some competition among us to stand out and get noticed. I found myself checking out the other waitresses constantly, jealous of their assets and the attention I thought it brought them, and it did my self-confidence no favors. Little blips of insecurity would pop up. I caught myself wishing my body were different and even contemplated straightening my hair, something I'd never even thought about before! I was so busy comparing myself that it stopped occurring to me that the 'fro made me stand out in a special way.

Then one day, the waitress that I considered to be the hottest of the group— she was dripping with sexual magnetism—gave me a compliment that made me see how blocked off I had become from my self-love. It was Halloween, and I came to work dressed as Wonder Woman. My juicy backside was hard to miss in that distinctive shiny leotard and those fishnets. She turned to me out of the blue and said, "Damn, girl, I would kill to have a butt like yours!" Until that moment, I'd just been jealous of her teeny, size 2 rear end. But then I looked at her, really looked, and I thought, *Yeah, we're both really sexy, just different.* (My extra ten pounds went to a good place!) I stopped comparing myself to other women right then and there.

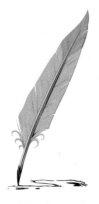

**JOURNALING
EXERCISE**

Write off the Jealousy!

Whether we like to admit it, we all have insecurities that can lead to resentment toward other women. In this exercise I want you to turn that negativity around. Write down five things that make you jealous of other women. Then, I want you to write what you could learn from them. Is it really her hair that men love or the way she flips it? Is it her small waist or the chic way she accessorizes it? Maybe she gets a lot of attention . . . because she is a master flirter? Then ask yourself, could you do the same or put your own twist on "her" moves? I know you can! So turn those *I can't do it*s into a *things to try* list and test them out this week. You'll look at yourself and other women in a different, positive light.

The big problem with comparing yourself to other women is that it diminishes your unique sexiness. And somehow, it always winds up breeding even more of this bad behavior. You can bet that while you're comparing yourself to someone across the room, they're comparing themselves to someone else. I'm here to tell you right now that this jealousy we all extend toward others has to stop for the good of all womankind! I want you to learn how to embrace not just your own sexiness but the sexiness of *all* women, and let it fuel your own Mojo. Once we acknowledge and identify with other women's Mojos, we can use that energy for a greater good—namely, helping to boost the Mojo of women who need it. We'll be unstoppable! So grab your pen again—let's work this one through!

3. LOOK FOR VISUAL AND MENTAL STIMULATION EVERY DAY

The more tuned in to yourself that you become, the more you start noticing that little tingle that appears when something starts to turn you on. Sure, all of us get our motors revved at the sight of a sexy scene in our favorite TV shows or when we think about past dalliances that really rocked our world. But there are seductive elements in *so* many places, you just need to keep your eyes open for them and embrace the opportunities they present. It could be a spectacularly phallic carrot, zucchini, or other natural wonder, or the way an orchid bloom resembles lady parts, even the way the air in the woods smells after it rains . . . musky, like sex.

I see sexy everywhere, and the women I've coached find they can, too. It's a mind-set, and once you've trained yourself to go there, the titillation all around becomes evident. (We often consider that men think about sex all the time, so why not us?) Working on this is one of the best ways to get sex on the front burners of your brain and feel frisky more often.

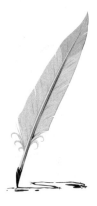

**JOURNALING
EXERCISE**

List Your *Daily Turn-ons!*

Get yourself a little notebook that you can carry along with you throughout your day (or tote your journal or just use an app on your phone) and make notes on the things that you see, hear, smell, and feel that please you and make you a little lusty. It could be anything from the words on a sign to a piece of art, the taste of strawberries on your tongue, a hot stranger wiping sweat from his forehead, the sensation of being touched by a stranger in a crowded elevator, or the sight of yourself in a lingerie fitting room. Remember, there are no wrong answers on this one; if it gives you a tingle, jot it down—even if it's not something you think "should" turn you on. And keep at it! The more you do this, the more it will help you identify what revs *your* motor.

4. LET GO OF SEX GUILT

We know that sex guilt can rob you of your Mojo, but it can also needlessly increase your stress level, decrease your self-esteem, and make you shut down where you should be opening up, which can hold you back from creating the sexiest lifestyle you've been dreaming of.

We all have different sexual histories, and sex guilt comes in many different forms and fashions. Not all of us have traumatic sexual experiences to work through, but there are other ways sex guilt can manifest itself. For example, is there anything you did in your past that makes you cringe or feel embarrassment? That counts, too. My hope is that through reflection you'll not only realize that these moments were part of your sexual education but that looking at them in a different light will help you let them go with forgiveness.

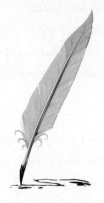

JOURNALING EXERCISE

Dwell on the *Past* for a Moment

Take a quiet moment out for yourself, and as honestly as you can, answer the questions below. It may feel like a challenge to unearth this stuff, but once you start to look at the not-so-hot experiences that you're still carrying with you, it will become easier to resolve them and push forward in your sexy transformation!

💜 What's your earliest memory of feeling guilty, shameful, confused, or embarrassed about sex?

💜 Has someone or something taught you to feel guilty about sex? How so?

💜 How do those situations resonate with you now?

💜 How have they hindered you from living your fullest, freest sex life possible?

💜 What would you do differently now that you have a different perspective on the situations?

💜 Can you find forgiveness for yourself, and extend it toward the situations?

💜 What can you do to make peace with them and let them go?

5. REVERSE NEGATIVE
BODY BANTER

Before we get to this exercise, I want to share a story with you. Back in 2001, I was going through a dark time in New York, where business was bad and boyfriends were worse . . . and I started to turn against my body, again. I was at a normal, healthy weight, but I became fixated on my thighs. I was lonely, couldn't find love, and was having a dry spell with sex—both with others and myself. I wasn't seeing myself in a beautiful way.

I remember standing in front of the mirror in my undies and hearing my inner voice literally attacking my thighs, saying, *You're so round! Why can't you be smaller? Why are you so big?* I was grabbing my outer thigh with my hand and wondering what my leg would look like if I had liposuction. It was as if the anxiety and uncertainty I was feeling about life was narrowing in on a body part. And that negative voice kept getting louder.

All of the sudden, I realized what I was doing to myself and it seemed *crazy!* Suddenly, the confident self-loving Dana that I'd cultivated my whole life was fed up. I marched myself into the bathroom and parked myself in front of the mirror. I looked deep into my own eyes and started saying out loud, *You're okay. You're beautiful. I love you. Stop this self-destructive nonsense. You're stronger than that. You love yourself way more than this!*

Over and over, I began saying affirmations of self-love. I was talking to myself the way I'd talk to my best friend in crisis. As days went on, I started incorporating dramatic grand affirmations like, *Thighs, you are terribly gorgeous. I love how juicy you are.* At first, it felt a little uncomfortable and sometimes utterly ridiculous. But that deep eye connection in the mirror was a major awakening for me. It was self-care in its purest form, and it was really when I turned away from negative body banter.

Now that mirror work has grown into something so far beyond the acute fix that I needed that day and into such a beautiful relationship that I have with myself. I truly love myself, and I love myself more every time I tell myself so! And this frees me up from dwelling on something that *truly* doesn't affect my inner light and my unique sexiness. Instead, I focus on what *is* feeling sexy and give myself a little bit of love. Once I started loving my body again, I started feeling sexier and happier, and that led me to finding happiness, sex, and love again!

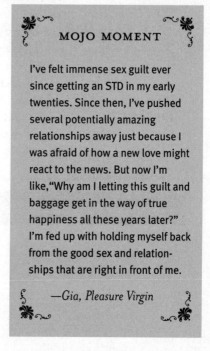

MOJO MOMENT

I've felt immense sex guilt ever since getting an STD in my early twenties. Since then, I've pushed several potentially amazing relationships away just because I was afraid of how a new love might react to the news. But now I'm like, "Why am I letting this guilt and baggage get in the way of true happiness all these years later?" I'm fed up with holding myself back from the good sex and relation-ships that are right in front of me.

—*Gia, Pleasure Virgin*

The worst thing about negative body banter is that it holds you back from fully enjoying sex and putting yourself out there to get it! If you don't bolster yourself up and adore every part of your body at every stage in your life, how can someone else?

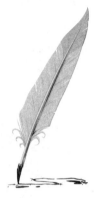

**JOURNALING
EXERCISE**

Time for Some
Positive Body Banter

This will teach you how to transform the negative messages you send yourself into more loving ones. Read the examples below and notice how each negative can be counteracted with a positive, sexy self-love saying. Then, I want you to write down some of the awful things you say to and about yourself, and flip them around to say something loving instead. Stand in the mirror, honey, look at yourself, and do as I did. That way you're building yourself up instead of tearing yourself down—and that's what's going to help you build your sexy self-confidence!

NEGATIVE BODY BANTER	SEXY SELF-LOVE SAYING
My thighs and ass are gigantic.	Look at those juicy buns and those deliciously curvy legs! Gorgeous!
I think my face is round, swollen, and fat.	My eyes are sparkling, my smile is electric, and I'm going to use them to captivate people!
I've got ten pounds of baby weight left over and I can't get rid of it. I hate it!	My body is incredible and magical and created the most amazing baby! If I can do that, I can do anything.

NEGATIVE BODY BANTER	SEXY SELF-LOVE SAYING
Why would anyone want to be with *this* body?	I'm super sexy, and dammit, I'm worth being desired!
I'm hesitant to take my clothes off in the bedroom—I don't want him to see my huge butt, boobs, thighs, tummy stretch marks, etc. I'm not relaxed enough.	I'm gonna rock my way into the bedroom with confidence— I deserve to be worshipped! Forget this hesitation, I'm making room for some sexy satisfaction!
IT'S YOUR TURN . . .	ADD YOUR OWN THOUGHTS!

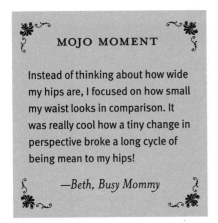

MOJO MOMENT

Instead of thinking about how wide my hips are, I focused on how small my waist looks in comparison. It was really cool how a tiny change in perspective broke a long cycle of being mean to my hips!

—*Beth, Busy Mommy*

Now take a little time to relax and absorb the things you've learned. You might be thinking, *Okay, I wrote down nice things about myself, but I still think my thighs are too round!* And that's okay—this is a process. You need to remind yourself every single day that you've been too hard on your beauty, your body, your sexual confidence . . . and yourself in general. It may take time, but if you don't start the journey, you'll never get anywhere. Negative body banter is a trap we all fall into sometimes, but the good news is that being aware of it is half the battle, and a solid step forward on your journey. We'll tackle more malfunctions as we move ahead.

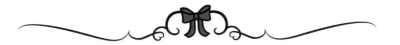

THE NEXT CHAPTER IS ALL ABOUT GETTING SEXY ON YOUR BRAIN (IN WAYS THAT ARE SO OBVIOUS, BUT SO EASY TO OVERLOOK): BY CARING FOR YOURSELF! YOU SHOULD BE DOING THIS ON A DAILY BASIS BUT CHANCES ARE YOU'RE NOT. LUCKILY, IT'S A HABIT THAT'S EASY TO ADOPT. THE PAYOFF IS IMMEDIATE BOTH IN HOW YOU LOOK AND FEEL ABOUT YOURSELF. IT'S TIME TO PRIMP.

CHAPTER SIX

Creating Seductive Beauty and Body Rituals

BEFORE YOU CAN LOVE SHARING YOUR BODY WITH A PARTNER OF your choosing, first you need to learn how to love that body yourself! Remember how I keep saying that confidence is the sexiest thing you can have? Creating seductive beauty and body rituals is one of the most powerful tools you have for buffing up your sexy self-confidence. And remember, not only will you feel better when you're lit up with confidence, you'll attract all kinds of positive attention from others, too!

These rituals are a chance for you to flirt with yourself, meditate in the mirror, and have simple sexy fun, girly style. And when you bask in this air of self-made bliss, you'll find your whole world begins to change in a sexier, more enchanted way.

So let go of the idea that your beauty routine is *routine*. From now on it's your sexy secret weapon!

GETTING STARTED

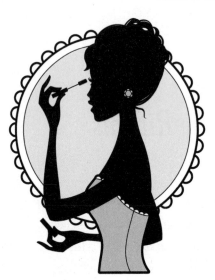

Okay, so what exactly is a seductive beauty ritual? It's an experience that transforms your daily self-care into something far more special—into an experience that becomes meaningful to your Mojo, your sexuality, femininity, confidence, and creativity. It's when you choose to use your makeup to unlock your inner vixen . . . when your morning application of body butter paves the road to accepting your thighs just as they are.

Step 1: Explore your beauty from the neck up

It doesn't matter what Mojo Model you are or what phase of life you're in. I know there's a whole lotta sexy about you, but we need to make sure *you* know it, too.

Focusing in on your sexiest beauty assets will help you create seductive beauty rituals around them, which will give you the confidence to step into the spotlight a little bit more. In turn, the parts you aren't as crazy about will take a backseat.

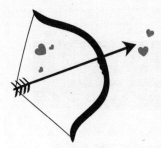

Creating *Seductive Beauty Rituals from the Neck Up*

Every day, when you do your morning and evening beauty routines, follow this exercise to transform that experience into a seductive beauty ritual. These work for even the most simple beauty routines!

EXERCISE

First, find the mirror in your home that you love best (you know, the one that has the most flattering lighting). Then continue using whatever makeup and hair products you usually would, but as you apply your eyeliner or mascara, blush, gloss, and spray, think sexier thoughts using the prompts below. Feel free to add more steps and thoughts into the blank spaces at the end of the chart.

FOCUS ON YOUR ASSETS (Don't be modest—the more the better!)	MAKE THEM TURN YOU ON (These easy moves feed your Mojo, big-time.)
YOUR EYES Are they large? Almond shaped? Do they "laugh" when you laugh? Do you have traffic-stopping eye color? Or fiery flecked color that makes your eyes magnetic? How about long lashes? Thick lashes? Sexy, flirty brows? Any of these will convey a sense of "come and get it!"	**SEDUCTIVE EYES RITUAL** Gaze into a mirror and imagine you're looking into the eyes of a lover, but turn that lust onto yourself! Lower your lids a bit, and tilt your head slightly up and down; raise a brow seductively, never breaking eye contact. Can you see how sexy you are?

FOCUS ON YOUR ASSETS (Don't be modest—the more the better!)	MAKE THEM TURN YOU ON (These easy moves feed your Mojo, big-time.)

YOUR LIPS

Are your lips soft and smooth? Full? Balanced? Do the corners curl up slyly when you smile or when you're thinking naughty thoughts? When you smile, do you beam that happiness so prettily and powerfully that it affects everyone around you? Make no mistake—your mouth can be magic.

SEDUCTIVE LIPS RITUAL

Strike a seductive pose: practice pursing your lips, just a hint, as you slightly lift your chin and open your lips a little bit, as if you're ready to be kissed. (Or maybe it's an expression of receiving others' pleasures— think like a porn star!) Gazing at those irresistible lips will make you *want* yourself!

YOUR CHEEKS

Think of how gorgeous they look when they're flushed with color—especially after a mind-blowing orgasm!—or how they frame your smile when you're really showing off your joy. If you haven't been playing them up, maybe you should!

SEDUCTIVE CHEEK RITUAL

There's no stopping the rush of blood during arousal. It's a raw reaction, and the way it tints your skin is h-o-t! Pinch your cheeks to bring the color into them. Right after that, your skin will have a peachy pink O-glow—a reminder of sizzling good times. Then, blend a hint of cream blush into the apples to keep that rush of sheer color all day long. Remember to think naughty thoughts!

FOCUS ON YOUR ASSETS
(Don't be modest—the
more the better!)

MAKE THEM TURN YOU ON
(These easy moves feed
your Mojo, big-time.)

YOUR HAIR

Sometimes we forget how hair can be a seductive tool. Is it shiny and healthy? Both things convey youthfulness and robust sexual health. Does it feel good to run your hands through it? Is it wavy like the hair of a statue of Venus? Or molten-lava straight like Jessica Rabbit's?

SEDUCTIVE HAIR RITUAL

While you're brushing your hair, imagine yourself in bed, titillating your lover with the sensation of your locks against his skin. At the same time fantasize a slo-mo movie movement: tossing your hair in a moment of passion. Go on, and give your hair a toss, a seductive flip. It will give your body's sexy centers a happy buzz.

NOW ADD MORE ASSETS . . .

. . . AND RITUALS OF YOUR OWN!

❤ After you've done this for a few days, write in your journal about the experience! How did it make you feel? Did you connect with yourself in a sexier way? If so, did the feelings stay with you as you went about your day? When you refreshed your lip gloss, did you remember the seductive feelings you created earlier on?

MOJO MEMO:

Compliment Your Beauty

I want you to give yourself a compliment every time you glance at yourself during the day. Because allowing yourself to revel in what's gorgeous about you will retrain your brain, teach you to see the beauty that you have, and to work it! Before you know it, you'll see only sexiness with every glance in the mirror.

Don't Just Apply Makeup— Seduce with It!

A well-placed dash of color can put a sexy spotlight on your favorite facial feature and really let it shine (and in turn, let you shine). Make these confidence-building beauty tips part of your A.M. and P.M. get-ready routines.

❤ **TRY SMOKY EYES.** Nothing draws attention to eyes like this timeless seductive look. The classic smoky eye is done by lining the eyes with dark eyeliner, topping it with matching shadow, and then fading the shadow upward on the lid to create a smudgy, just-had-a-sex-romp look. For daytime, choose medium-depth colors like cocoa, bronze, copper, purple, and forest green. Lining the top lid only may be enough "smoke" for day, especially for smaller or round eyes. But do experiment with a more daring all-around lining job, especially if you have large or almond-shaped eyes. At night choose a deep vixen-vibe shade like charcoal, black, deep eggplant, or midnight navy. And don't forget the black mascara—one coat for daytime and two at night.

❤ **PLUMP-IFY YOUR PUCKER.** Lovely, lusciously sheer colors make your lips look juicy and irresistible to boot! One of my favorite Booty Parlor products is called Kissaholic—it's an aphrodisiac-infused pout-plumping lip gloss that makes your lips feel sexy and spicy all at once, with exotic ingredients designed to inspire desire! Whatever brand of gloss you choose, try one in red or berry. They'll mimic the deep natural hue your lips get after a long makeout session.

❤ **GET AN R-RATED FLUSH.** Blush's whole purpose is to mimic the youthful flush that signals fertility and sexuality. (Think of Scarlett O'Hara pinching her cheeks as she prepped to seduce Rhett Butler.) Choose a creamy formula instead of a powder. Why? The nonmatte finish will leave your skin looking dewy, the way it does after a steamy sex marathon!

❤ **LET YOUR MANE FLOW WILD!** Fantasies abound about the buttoned-up secretary who unleashes her hair and becomes a wanton sex goddess, and there's a reason—it's hot! Try it yourself. Start the show by pulling your tresses into a sexy bun or ponytail. If your hair is shorter, slide it off your face with a chic headband. When the time's right, let your partner see you release your hair—make sure to play it up with lots of flipping and tossing. That moment of letting go can be a super sexy preview of what's ahead, for you both!

Step 2: Explore your assets from the neck down

It's time to focus your attention downward and pay some loving attention to that gorgeous bod! After you give yourself the time and care to address your beautiful assets, I'm going to give you one ritual that worships the whole neck-to-toe package at once. To start, strip down and check yourself out in a full-length mirror. Dress scantily—maybe in a bra and panties or better yet, nothing at all. Do this after you've showered, with freshly shaved legs and well-lubricated skin because you'll feel your sexy best when your bod is all soft and glowing.

Ready? Start complimenting your feminine curves. I know there are positives, and I want you to see them, too.

- ♥ **Neck, shoulders, and collarbone.** These are universally erogenous parts—a mere whisper of breath on them can get your blood pumping. With a fingertip, trace the curves and contours and take pleasure in the way the smooth, soft skin reacts to your touch.

- ♥ **Bust.** Big, small, there's room for them all! Large and round, small and perfectly proportioned to your frame. Be sure to give props to your nipples; they're at the core of feminine beauty and a pleasure point, too.

- ♥ **Tummy.** A sexy stomach, whether it's a tight firm washboard; a kissably soft tummy accentuated by a nipped-in waist and jaw-dropping hip curves; or a tummy adorned with a darling belly button; they all deserve attention (so love yours just as it is).

- ♥ **Buns.** As with boobs, bodacious booties come in all shapes. Tight, juicy, petite, ample. Pay homage to your special shape with a rowdy double hand slap—on bare skin, of course!

- ♥ **Legs.** There's nothing like a great pair of gams, and they come in all sorts of shapes and sizes, too! Thighs that can grip a partner and ride hard are worth showing off. Lean legs can slide into any jeans (like skinny jeans, my personal nemesis). Knees can be naturally sexy or made to look that way in sky-high heels. The curve of a muscular calf is titillating and something no starving supermodel can boast. And let's not forget the joys of beautifully shaped sexy feet with toes that beg to be kissed.

YOUR SEDUCTIVE BODY RITUAL

Your new, body-encompassing ritual will go something like this. After you've finished toweling off that sexy bod, reach for your cream of choice. Whatever your preference may be, choose something that smells delicious and makes you excited to put all over your body.

As you're taking your time to delicately caress lotion into your skin, use the moment to worship yourself. Tell yourself how much you love the strong curve of your calf as your hands glide over it, how you're appreciative of your tummy and all that it does, and how desirable and feminine your breasts, hips, buns, and thighs are. Everywhere you have a curve, you should be giving it loving attention! You might even consider getting a glamorous powder puff and dusting your curves with shimmer powder to finish off the ritual. (If it has a yummy, edible taste, even better!)

Though it may feel strange at first, I promise you, the more you do this, the more you're going to fall in love with yourself. I encourage you to do this anytime, but especially when you're feeling like your ass is extra huge, or your muffin top spilleth over. Instead of focusing on the negative, grab hold of your body and tell it how much you love it!

ANOTHER MUST:
CREATE A SEDUCTIVE BATH RITUAL

Another way to adore your whole body is to submerge it. Often we're in such a rush with our beauty rituals that we opt for quick showers, and forget about the seductive experience of having a bath. The bathtub is a phenomenal place to escape from the world (or just someone else in your house), to release life's cares, and to get in touch with your relaxed sexy self. If you haven't been taking at least a half-hour out of your week to take part in one, you're missing out . . . and it's about time you tuned into the tub. Creating a seductive bath ritual can be a very inspiring experience, both on a sexy self-care and a Mojo-boosting level. Here are my suggestions:

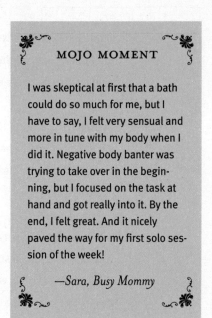

MOJO MOMENT

I was skeptical at first that a bath could do so much for me, but I have to say, I felt very sensual and more in tune with my body when I did it. Negative body banter was trying to take over in the beginning, but I focused on the task at hand and got really into it. By the end, I felt great. And it nicely paved the way for my first solo session of the week!

—*Sara, Busy Mommy*

❤ **Choose music.** While you're running your bath, pick some tunes that help you unwind, like something slow and sultry to get you in a sexy mood.

❤ **Dress your bath.** Don't forget to add tasty treats to your tub! Of course, I recommend Booty Parlor's Naughty Bubbles or our luxuriantly moisturizing Bath Milk, but you can always use your favorite bubble bath, bath bombs, or even some essential oils like lavender or sweet orange.

♥ **Light some candles.** Nothing ruins the solitude of a bath like bright overhead lighting. Flip the switches off and use candles to help create a sensual mood.

♥ **Reserve your unwind time.** Close the door, make sure everyone knows you're not to be disturbed (or better, plan ahead for a time when you're home alone), and let yourself melt into the cocoon of warm water.

♥ **Don't forget those curves!** When you're nice and calm, massage your lovely legs, awesome arms, and everything in between with a decadent lathering wash and a luxuriously soft sponge. And if it inspires you to have a sexy solo session, even better!

LET'S GET PHYSICAL!

Of course, you're aware of the health benefits of exercise, but are you clued into how much of a Mojo booster working out is? It's true! Once those little endorphins go racing around in you, your inner spark gets nurtured in a way that can't be denied. No question, exercise can help you feel more in control of your body, more in touch with the power of your body, and more excited to show it off—to yourself or someone else.

Choosing workouts that boost your sexual fitness

Whether you have a set fitness routine or not, I want you to open your mind to allow in some different workouts. Because I want you to think about *sexy fitness*. What's that? When I say sexy fitness, I mean, classes that tune you into your female body and mind and your Mojo. Sexy fitness is not about burning calories on a spin bike. It's about workouts with a sensual underbelly that create awareness of your parts and how you move them. Keep an eye out for exotic-dance classes like pole dancing, burlesque, Latin or African dance, or even Zumba (the hip gyrations that are a core part of the class are just like the moves you use when you're on your partner). I've even seen classes on how to walk in exotic high-heeled shoes. You can download full workouts at iTunes or short free ones on YouTube. But try to do one at a gym or an all-female fitness center. I love working out with other women because the rawness of glistening curves, heavy

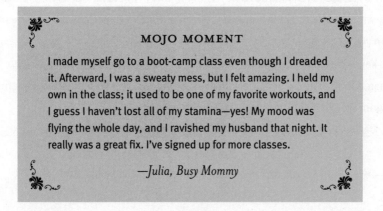

MOJO MOMENT

I made myself go to a boot-camp class even though I dreaded it. Afterward, I was a sweaty mess, but I felt amazing. I held my own in the class; it used to be one of my favorite workouts, and I guess I haven't lost all of my stamina—yes! My mood was flying the whole day, and I ravished my husband that night. It really was a great fix. I've signed up for more classes.

—Julia, Busy Mommy

breathing, and girl-tastic vitality all around me is electric. In order to embrace your body's beauty, you need to appreciate it in other women, too: feminine bodies in all different gorgeous shapes, from toned hotties to softer foxes.

YOUR FITNESS RITUAL: I want you to commit to doing one seductive fitness activity a week, whether it's a class or a video. Better yet, invite a group of girls to experience it with you, and then compare notes afterward about how you could apply the moves to a sexy romp.

A Mojo must: the O workout!

Strengthening the pelvic floor muscles (also called pubococcygeus muscles, or PC muscles for short) can help boost your orgasms, both in intensity and frequency. That's because squeezing the muscles increases blood flow to your lady parts, which can increase pleasurable sensations. That, in turn, is a major confidence booster. They also help you grip onto him, which will drive him wild! And if you're single, you'll grip your toys more firmly, which will drive you wilder!

All it takes is ten minutes a day. And the way I look at it, that's ten minutes a day when you're thinking about sex, which goes a long way to wanting more of it with yourself, and others!

Kegel exercises (named for Arnold Kegel, the renowned gynecologist who created them) can be done on your own, or you can give your muscles something to grip onto by inserting a vaginal (V-Spot) barbell.

Okay—ready to get a stronger V-Spot? Here's how to Kegel like a pro:

❤ **Find your orgasm muscles.** Next time you're peeing, stop yourself midstream—the muscles that stop the flow are your PC muscles.

(PC muscles are also responsible for the contractions you feel in an orgasm—that's the link!)

💜 **Practice contracting them.** The basic pee-halting motion is one Kegel. Once you have the motion down pat, don't make a habit of doing it while you pee; doing so can actually weaken the muscles over time.

💜 **Practice holding them.** Hold one Kegel for three seconds, followed by a three-second rest. Repeat ten times for one set. Do three sets every day.

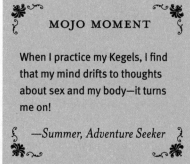

MOJO MOMENT

When I practice my Kegels, I find that my mind drifts to thoughts about sex and my body—it turns me on!

—Summer, Adventure Seeker

💜 **Step it up a notch!** Once three-second holds become easier, switch to four-second holds and four-second rests. Work up to ten-second holds with ten-second rests. And remember to perform three sets of ten holds three times a day. For even more fun, add workout music to help get you pumped!

💜 **Heat up your sessions with naughty thoughts.** Envisioning yourself as a stronger sexual being (literally) will help harness your sexual energy and charge up your Mojo.

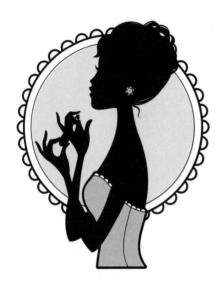

EAU YES!
USING FRAGRANCE TO FEEL SEXY

Scent is such an incredible part of our lives. We often forget how powerful the sense of smell can be when it comes to sexual attraction. It's not just an important part of attracting others, it's important in seducing yourself! You're about to learn how to use scent to your best steamy advantage.

There's no question that a scent can trigger specific memories about a person, place, or time. If there was a sexual buzz surrounding the way you experienced an aroma, you can revisit that confidence-boosting Mojo again just as powerfully by smelling it again. But to get the benefits, you'll need to find out what works best for you.

How to find your own seductive scent

Finding the smells that snap your brain into lusty mode is easy. Just follow these steps!

♥ **Write down aromas that make you swoon.** Connect your sexiest memories to a time and place where they happened, and you'll probably find a scent association. Maybe it's lilacs because you stood near them for your first meaningful kiss, or maybe you got busy in a fruit orchard, at the beach, in the woods . . . You get the idea. Foods count here, too, because we smell what we eat. So include chocolate mousse, apricot tart, spices (like from that Thai restaurant where you met a lover) if that's where your memories guide you.

♥ **Take it online.** The Fragrance Foundation's Web site, Fragrance .org, is a great resource because you can see what perfumes have the aroma notes on your list. Jot down a handful of perfumes you think you'll like and take the list to a store.

♥ **Inhale.** Test your scents on plain paper. It will help you to narrow down the options to a few that you can then try on your skin. (If you like it on paper, you'll like it on your skin.) The right sexy scent will elicit a visceral reaction—you'll *feel* turned on.

SEDUCTIVE SCENT RITUAL: To build anticipation for a solo session later that day, dab your sexy scent onto your inner thighs only and pull on a pair of pants to keep it under wraps. The scent will lay dormant until you get naked and start heating things up for yourself. As your thighs rub while your solo session heats up, the aroma will be released. As you inhale deeply and quickly with every O pulsation, your olfactory nerves will be washed over with the seductive scent, waking up parts of your brain. Then try it with a skirt on a warm day . . . the scent will rise up while you're on the go and give your brain something pleasant to think about.

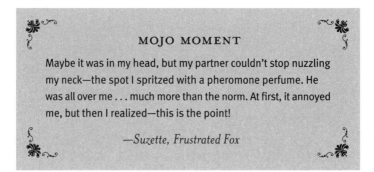

MOJO MOMENT

Maybe it was in my head, but my partner couldn't stop nuzzling my neck—the spot I spritzed with a pheromone perfume. He was all over me . . . much more than the norm. At first, it annoyed me, but then I realized—this is the point!

—Suzette, Frustrated Fox

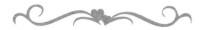

USING SCENT
IN THE BEDROOM

Scent your bedroom (or any room—even your car) with a fragrance you associate with orgasmic delight. Smelling it will make you want to get your groove on. Experiment with candles (imagine the jumping flame is your C-Spot), or purchase a laundry wash or dryer sachet in a fragrance you groove on and use it to scent your linens. Essential oils can be drizzled onto a quilted cotton makeup pad or a tissue and tucked into your pillowcases, or they can be used in oil burners that release scent gently into the air. Test different options to find the mode that gives you the most pleasure.

PHEROMONES:
YOUR FLIRTY LITTLE
SECRET

Now that you've got a scent that incites lusty feelings, let's talk about adding another sexy secret weapon into the mix—sex pheromones! These are natural chemicals secreted by animals (humans included!), plants, and insects to attract and hook up with mates. They work like invisible attraction agents that make you irresistible to others and help boost your confidence sky-high! That's why I worked to create products in the Booty Parlor line that use pheromones as part of their

formula makeup. Try a pheromone-laced perfume instead of your signature one and dab it on a few sexy spots, like below your belly button, right where the lower back curves into your buttocks, and on your ankles. Think of it like an Easter egg hunt. As your partner explores your body and his olfactory nerves register the pheromones, they'll elicit an intense reaction that he'll forever associate with you. He won't know what hit him!

ANYTIME ACTIVITY: SEXY BEAUTY AND BODY RITUAL AFFIRMATIONS

A huge part of your sexy beauty rituals is using affirmations to help you make a solid connection to loving your beautiful sensual self and help you to boost your sexy self-confidence as you're preparing for your day. It's okay if you're not sure how to do

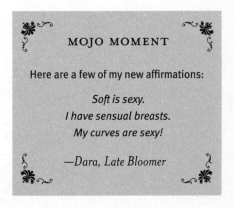

MOJO MOMENT

Here are a few of my new affirmations:

Soft is sexy.
I have sensual breasts.
My curves are sexy!

—*Dara, Late Bloomer*

this. Below, I've shared some of my favorites to help you get started. Use them to inspire you to create some of your own sexy self-confidence!

💜 My eyes have a beautiful color that's intense and mesmerizing.

💜 I have luscious, kissable lips that are ready to receive and give pleasure.

💜   I have strong, sexy curves in my legs, from my thighs all the way down to my calves. They're powerful and womanly, which I love!

💜   I adore my luscious tummy, and how it feels to glide my hands across it, touching every soft contour it has to share.

💜   I'm head over heels for my juicy butt! It's firm and full, and oh so grab-able!

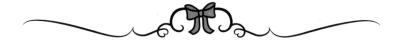

KEEP UP THE GOOD RITUALS!

THE MORE YOU WORK WITH YOUR SEXY RITUALS ON ALL LEVELS, THE MORE YOU'RE GOING TO COME INTO YOUR FABULOUS FLIRTY SELF AND TRULY OWN THE STUNNING CREATURE THAT YOU ARE. AND JUST LIKE WITH ANY RELATIONSHIP, MAKE SURE YOUR RITUALS DON'T GET STALE. MIX THEM UP, INVENT NEW THINGS TO SAY AND DO, AND SEE HOW MUCH FURTHER YOU CAN TAKE THEM ON YOUR OWN!

This Week's Mojo Mission

INFUSE EVERY DAY WITH SEX APPEAL

It's time to get busy bringing sexy into your life on a daily basis. You'll lean on your best friends here because there's nothing like a girl group to cheer you on (or nudge you along, if that's what it takes!). You'll also learn how to express your budding Mojo through new changes to your wardrobe and bedroom.

GET READY TO

- ♥ Get your girls together and talk about sex and sexiness!

- ♥ Learn how to dress the part for a more confident, sexier lifestyle.

- ♥ Turn your bedroom into a seductive sanctuary.

KEEP UP THE GOOD MOJO WORK!

Valuing yourself as a sexy, beautiful, deserving woman is tied in closely with self-care. So continue to make beauty and body rituals a regular part of your weekly routine. This will help keep a stream of sexy thoughts floating through your mind!

CHAPTER SEVEN

Let's Talk About Sex, Girls!

YOUR LOVER ISN'T THE ONLY ONE YOU SHOULD BE SHARING YOUR desires with. As part of your makeover, I want you to engage in frisky, honest, and frequent sex chats with your gal pals. Talking with your girlfriends about sex keeps you mentally focused on your Mojo and creates a safe supportive forum to share your boudoir triumphs and tribulations, develop (and exchange) your repertoire of sexy tips and tricks, and help give you sexy ammo for upcoming sessions with your partner!

INITIATING REGULAR GIRLS' NIGHT SEX-TALK SESSIONS

As far as I'm concerned, regular girls' nights are a must. They are my saving grace, my lifeline, my reason to leave the office exactly on time that day. My girlfriends lift my spirit, keep me in check, and listen to my endless ramblings. I feel safe enough to share my deepest secrets and to air out my insecurities and fears. I love the honesty, the camaraderie, the confidence boosting, the clothes swapping, and the wine swigging. But perhaps what I love the most about getting together for girls' night (which is almost always on Tuesday) are the conversations we have about sex.

We talk about everything related to sex. What we're doing, whom we're doing it with (half my gang is single; half is married), what's turning us on, what new things we're trying. Nothing is off topic—sizes and shapes, sexual positions, the bedroom accessories we're using (usually this winds up with me whipping out and discussing a new contraption I received at work!). We talk about our orgasms and our lady bits, including our sexual health, grooming habits, and the way our cycles affect our sex drives. We reveal our secret sexual fantasies and share our best sex tips and tricks. It's not all about the amazing sex we're having, because let's face it—sex isn't always amazing. We use girls' night to share the real problems we experience in the bedroom (and our relationships). We may not always find the solutions to our problems, but having the safe and nurturing space a girls' night offers gives us the perfect forum to be open and honest. And that can go a long way toward helping each of us feel as if we have broader sexual perspectives and fresh takes on how to move through the issues. It's a Mojo boost all around!

Kick off your girls' night!

Now it's time for you to organize a girls' night of your own, with a special focus: a girls' night sex-chat session. Pulling it together is blissfully simple.

INVITE THE RIGHT GROUP. Choose a small group of girlfriends (four's a good number) that you already feel very open and free with, and all of whom feel comfortable and communicative around one another. Send out an e-mail (or create an Evite) that entices them with the promise of a fun and frisky evening of racy chatter!

SET THE SCENE. Even though it's just the ladies coming over, go ahead and set the scene for steamy conversation! Set out flowers, light candles, play some fun and flirty music, and create a signature cocktail for those who might need a little liquid courage (and those who don't, as well!). Think along the lines of a Mojo Mojito, Kissable Cosmo, Coquettish Colada, Seductive Seabreeze . . . there are some great online resources to help you find a good concoction.

ALLOW CHAT TIME. Though it's sex-talk night at your place, give your friends a moment to get comfortable before you leap into the main event. Once everyone is done venting about their days, they'll be loose enough to get down to the nitty-gritty!

MAKE LIKE LAS VEGAS. What happens at girls' night, stays at girls' night. Promising one another that everything divulged at girls' night will get locked in the vault adds that extra level of comfort and security, allowing each of your friends to really put it out there. This way, you can get to the really good stuff!

DO IT AGAIN! Chances are you and your friends will have laughed, learned, and grown so much that you'll want to make this a regular event. Suggest a host rotation so that everyone gets the chance to have the girls over—and run the evening in their own unique way which can allow for even more interesting, illuminating, and surprising sexy revelations!

TIPS FOR STARTING
THOSE LUSTY CONVERSATIONS

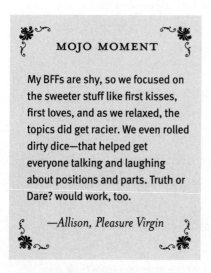

MOJO MOMENT

My BFFs are shy, so we focused on the sweeter stuff like first kisses, first loves, and as we relaxed, the topics did get racier. We even rolled dirty dice—that helped get everyone talking and laughing about positions and parts. Truth or Dare? would work, too.

—Allison, Pleasure Virgin

While attending regular girls' nights will help you become more and more comfortable talking about sex, you're in charge of this first soiree, so you'd better get prepared to lead the way! The tips below will definitely help get the raunchy chatter flowing.

Steamy starter topics

Having a list of themes will help you drive the conversations and will take the pressure off your guests to come up with the night's talking points (especially if some of your friends are shy). I suggest choosing two or three for each get-together and sending them ahead of time so everyone has a chance to prep their sexiest, silliest, and sultriest thoughts and stories to share that night—giving your girls time to get excited about what they're going to share will boost everyone's Mojo!

♥ **Firsts.** You can talk about your first kiss, your first solo session, your first PDA, your first one-night stand. It doesn't matter how tame or how wild, firsts can be great icebreakers—and they'll naturally take the conversation to seconds, thirds, bests, and favorites.

♥ **Sexy screen scenes.** When it comes to inspiring sexual fantasies, nothing does it quite like a steamy film scene—or a hot Hollywood actor who has starred in one. Share your faves, trade notes, and discover a new hunk (or new screen obsession!).

♥ **Toys and tools.** Are you a toy novice or an old pro? Do you have a favorite or one that you hoped would knock your socks off but didn't? Discussing toys and tools—both that you've used and haven't— can help open you up to sexy experiences you might not have known about or even deepen an experience you're already having.

♥ **Orgasms.** Whether you have them or not, orgasms are always a great topic of discussion. Discuss the best, the worst, the surprises, the disappointments, and the ones you have both with yourself as well as with someone else! What makes them unique, and how can you have more?

♥ **Sex flubs.** It's fun to talk about good sex, but talking about when bad sex happens can help you work through it in a way you might not have been able to on your own. You can share stories of techniques that didn't work, sizzling moments that fizzled, and what you desire from your partner but aren't getting. Most of all, this makes you feel that you're not alone: there's no perfect relationship, and bad sex happens, and that's okay. A little girlfriend-to-girlfriend advice on such things can help you find ways to turn things around.

These topics just scratch the surface! As you and the girls start talking, keep a mental list of other hot topics that come up, then jot them down in your journal so you don't forget.

GET IT GOING:
SCRIPTS TO GET YOU STARTED

Once you know the topic, it helps to have a monologue that allows you to welcome your girls and gives them a sense of where this can go. (Having structure also prevents topics from fizzling.) A well-prepared cheat sheet can help take your sex-chat session to new heights, drawing out interesting and insightful discoveries that you wouldn't have otherwise uncovered. Let's say your topic for the evening is *The Hottest Sex I Ever Had*. Here's how your lead-in might sound:

Tonight, we're going to talk about hot sex—those sizzling, lusty, uninhibited sexual experiences we've all had, the encounters that we still think about, that still turn us on even though they may have happened years ago with someone who's not our current lover, in another phase and time of our lives.

It may have been the wild one-night stand where you ripped each other's clothes off before you knew each other's names. The time you had sex in the freight elevator with your skirt hiked up. The spontaneous sex you had where you wound up conceiving your baby. The time you let him tie you up and surrendered to being completely ravished by him. The months of impulsive, decadent summer sex you had while backpacking through Europe in college. Get what I'm talking about? Unless one of you wants to jump in, I can start!

QUESTIONS TO START THE CONVERSATION

These will help get you started, but wait and see—as the conversations evolve (along with everyone's comfort levels), you'll find it becomes easier and easier to set the themes for each evening.

- ♥ What's the hottest sex you've ever had?

- ♥ What specifically made it so unforgettable? The lover? The location? Did you try something kinky?

- ♥ Have you ever secretly fantasized about a past lover while with your current one?

- ♥ Did it expand your capacity for amazing sex?

- ♥ Would you ever want to revisit that lover or experience if you could?

MOJO MOMENT

I'm so proud of myself. I went *way* out of my comfort zone and tried one of the scripts, and the girls totally responded the way I hoped. They even said it was hot to hear me read my cheat sheet out loud!

—*Allison, Pleasure Virgin*

Okay, it's your turn now. Decide the topic for your fist powwow and scribble down your lead-in to use as a cheat sheet (your friends won't care if you read it out loud). As your Mojo continues to magnify, you'll start thinking and talking about sex more often, and coming up with provocative topics and questions for your girls' nights will become second nature to you!

SWAPPING SEX TIPS
AND SEXY FANTASIES

Have you ever gone to a clothing-swap party with your girlfriends? Everyone leaves with something new to add to her wardrobe, and it didn't cost anyone a penny. Sounds fabulous, right? Well, I want you to take that same concept and spice it up, transforming one of your weekly girls' nights into a sex-tip swap!

How does it work? Pass around index cards and have your girls write down their top three sex tips. Explain that their tips could range from the sexual techniques that help them reach orgasm every time to recommendations on how they get in the mood, or even insights on a special spot that—when stimulated ever so softly—makes their lovers go crazy. But don't stop there. Instruct them to write down their top three sexual fantasies on the other side of the card. Think you knew your friends inside and out? This is where you may be surprised!

Once everyone has written their top three tips and fantasies, you have two options. First, go around the circle, sharing and discussing one tip at a time. Continue until you get through everyone's tips and then repeat the cycle with the fantasies. Alternatively, you could put the cards in a bowl, mix them up, and then pick one to read. The point is to pick someone's card other than your own. This adds another dimension to the discussion, and some anonymity until the group starts to figure out who wrote what, and discovers whose fantasies are the wildest, funniest, or dirtiest! Whichever way you choose to run the swap, every single one of your girlfriends will benefit.

They'll leave girls' night with an arsenal of sexy tips to try, and their imaginations will be fueled by the fantasies that were revealed, which may just spark up new some fantasies of their own!

You may find your friends say, "What do you mean, *write down a sex tip*? Like what?" Whether they say that or not, you'll want to give them some fodder to get started. Here are some prompts to talk through as you start the activity:

💜 **Solo tips.** Whether you're single or coupled up, sharing tips on your sexy solo sessions is always welcome! Have you learned of a new toy or bedroom accessory, or did you figure out a new, inventive, or surprising way to bring yourself to the Big O? Maybe there's just a move you've got that's so tried-and-true it'd be a crime against womankind if you don't share it!

💜 **Partner tips.** Who doesn't want to learn new tips to love your lover? Write down a position that blew your mind. Suggest ways to turn each other on, like reading erotic stories or surfing through sexy online videos. Or recommend a more adventurous encounter that you tried, and loved.

♥ **Flirting tips.** Flirting doesn't help you just nab your mate; it helps you keep him interested—and perhaps most important, keeps you feeling frisky, turned on, and tuned in to the power of your Mojo! Your flirting tips might involve a game of footsie, a foolproof winking technique, or the down-and-dirty verbal seduction that got you exactly what you wanted the other night.

♥ **Forbidden fantasies.** Nothing's off-limits here, so go wild and express yourself! Do you secretly dream of being dominated or dominating him? What about playing teacher and student? A threesome, sex with a stranger, voyeurism, maybe performing a sexy striptease? These may seem unrealistic or beyond your current sexual boundaries—but that's the point! They're fantasies! Let's reveal what secretly turns us on!

♥ **Celebrity fantasies.** Brad Pitt, Johnny Depp, George Clooney . . . yummy! There are so many to choose from. Sometimes nothing gets our Mojo rising quite like lusty thoughts of being entwined with our favorite Hollywood star, or two of them at once. Who's yours, and what's your fantasy? Don't skimp on the details!

♥ **Location fantasies.** Have you ever thought about having steamy sex on the beach? The middle of a forest with no one around for miles and miles? Elevators, airplanes, on top of a desk in his office? Where would you love to be seduced?

As you're going to discover with practice, the more you talk about sex with your girlies, the more you're going to boost your Mojo. It just has a way of boosting your confidence and making you feel bombshell bold. Plus, it will also better prepare you for communicating with your lover on your wants and needs. And guess what that does? You got it—boosts your Mojo even further! The more you find your footing and comfort level in talking openly about sex and your desires, the more capable you'll be at getting what you want. You'll have a better foundation to help you take control of your satisfaction. There's a lot of power involved with speaking up for what you desire. Once you harness that, it will change your whole life!

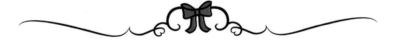

NO DOUBT, YOU'VE GOTTEN YOURSELF
ALL WORKED UP WITH ALL OF THIS
SEXY THINKING AND TALKING!
I HOPE IT WILL INSPIRE YOU IN THE NEXT CHAPTER.
ARE YOU READY TO MAKE OVER YOUR WARDROBE
AND LINGERIE DRAWER WITH SOME
SASSY, SEDUCTIVE PIECES? LET'S GO!

CHAPTER EIGHT

Sexy-up Your Wardrobe

L AST WEEK, YOU TOSSED OUT ALL THE HOLEY, OUTDATED, AND ill-fitting clothes that were doing your sexy self-confidence no favors, and now it's time to help you evolve your personal style a bit further. By this chapter's end, I want you to recognize that dressing to please yourself is a major Mojo booster and a pleasure you deserve daily. No question—figuring out your unique sexy style will take some thought. The quizzes here will help you identify the looks that will take you to a new level of sexiness but won't make you feel as though you're wearing someone else's version of sexy. And that's so important. As I've said before, how you *feel* in your clothes matters most—so if you're a sexy jock, a ruffled floral style won't feel right, and in turn, it won't give you a sexy self-confidence boost. Ready to set your style compass for hot?

UNDERSTANDING SEXY STYLE

So what is sexy style? It's about representing your sexiest self through clothes and accessories and about how you wrap it all together and work it. And to get there, you're trying lots of new things to see whether you like them and how they can work for you. If you don't try new things out—and new things on—you can't know what works. Sexy style is simply the representation of you, and if you're feeling strong and sexy and comfortable in your personal style (by comfortable, I mean, comfortable in your own skin), you'll feel confident. And of course, I'll say it again: confidence is the sexiest thing a woman can have—or wear, for that matter!

Your sexy style will grow and evolve, but so long as you're *allowing* it to grow and evolve, it can always be a source of sexiness for you and make you feel great about yourself. In college, my sexy style was about short skirts, layered tights with thigh-highs, and grungy fake-fur coats. That evolved into my beatnik phase of black turtlenecks and tight black leggings, always carrying a Jack Kerouac book or reciting poetry with my other beatnik

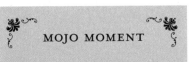

MOJO MOMENT

I have spectacular boobs (I got them in my twenties), and I love to show them off. But I had been focusing on my legs as part of my new bath ritual. They're pretty awesome, too. So I reversed my style for a night. I covered up a bit more on top and stepped out in a miniskirt. I felt like a different woman; it was weird in a good way. There's more to love in me than just my breasts.

—*Angela, Adventure Seeker*

friends. It was youth, it was pure freedom, and it was sexy. Later on, I discovered Diane von Furstenberg and landed on what will forever be a sexy go-to for me—the wrap dress. Any pattern, almost any color—put me in one and I immediately feel sexy, feminine, curvy, and delicious. During my pregnancy, my sexy style was tight leggings, long, tight tank tops to showcase my bump, sexy heels and a draping jersey cardigan to give me some rump coverage. I've found the balance where I can be comfy and sexy, and that definitely helps keep my Mojo powered up.

FINDING THE LOOKS
THAT BOOST YOUR MOJO

Defining your personal daily sexy style can be tough without some points of reference. It will help if you have a style identity to refer to. Think of this exercise as a turbo boost to help you navigate your closet, your dresser, and the local mall.

MOJO MEMO:

Check out H&M or Forever 21 if you have them near you—both stores organize clothes in ways that make pulling outfits together simple, and the wallet-friendly prices make it easy to load your closet with the styles that will boost your sexy self-confidence. Of course, there are also stores (like Anthropologie, J.Crew, or countless online boutiques) devoted to one style sensibility, which helps avoid having a mishmash of pieces that don't work together.

To help you pinpoint the looks that will enrich your Mojo—the wardrobe pieces you'll feel passionate about and will make you feel like a million bucks every day—first check your Mojo Motivation Board, then read through the style identities below and see which one speaks to you the loudest. With that archetype in mind as you shop in stores, you'll start to notice that clothes and accessories are typically merchandised in groups very much like these, which makes it easy to mix pieces that all hang together. You'll also see that I've included some sexy style suggestions to help make it easier to nail down those first few purchases. Don't forget, if budget is an issue, consider a clothing swap with your friends, as I mentioned earlier. They work!

Okay, get ready to find yourself!

1. *Contemporary Bohemian*

Think: Chloë Sevigny, Sienna Miller, Rachel Bilson. You love feminine, soft, vintage-inspired looks, and you're probably inclined to ground them with a great-fitting pair of jeans or pants. (The actress Chloë Sevigny has amazing legs, and if you do, too, look up her amazing boho-chic looks; she knows how to rock a mini and look like a modern hippie goddess.) Anthropologie is one of your dream stores, so look at their Web site for inspiration on how to layer clothes and accessories. *Sexy stockups for any day:* A billowy feminine top (with an ultraopen neck), paired with a chunky, layered necklace and a bauble ring; jeans and a cute leather satchel. Vintage-inspired handbags can have adorable embellishments like flower appliqués—but avoid anything too girlish. While it might be fun, it's not hot, and hot is your goal.

2. Feminine Frill Seeker

Scarlett Johansson and Eva Mendes are frilly
girls. Drew Barrymore's playful, whimsical
style touches qualify her. You gravitate
toward things that are lacy, embellished, and
romantic, like sweaters with ruffles or
multistrand-layered necklaces that combine
sheer fabric with a chain and gorgeous
beading. For a Saturday night out, you'd love
to see yourself in a printed matte jersey wrap

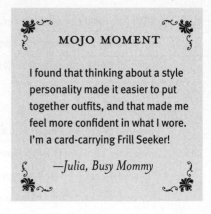

MOJO MOMENT

I found that thinking about a style
personality made it easier to put
together outfits, and that made me
feel more confident in what I wore.
I'm a card-carrying Frill Seeker!

—Julia, Busy Mommy

dress that shows off the girls just so, coupled with chandelier earrings or loads
of delicate charm necklaces. *Sexy stockups for any day:* A sheer lacy tunic to wear
with a cami over leggings, sexy heels, and a whimsically long necklace with
sensual glass droplets.

3. Modern Minimalist

Jennifer Lopez, Jennifer Aniston, Halle Berry. Understated but notably sexy,
elegance is where you want to be fashion-wise. You're drawn to clean, put-
together looks—you get excited by a chic sateen jacket that fits like a glove more
than you do a frilly sweater. Shift dresses; pencil skirts; military-inspired details,
like zippers and pockets; and basically anything in white, beige, or black are
things you make a beeline for when you shop. A dark flowing top with fitted
jeans and heels is how you'd like to dress for a Saturday night out. *Sexy stockups
for any day:* A solid-color silky blouse with a low-draped neck or other feminine

detail (that you can wear under your structured jackets and with black jeans or trousers), and shoes that combine a bit of an S-and-M vibe, like thick leather straps or brushed metallic accents, with a womanly stiletto heel.

4. Pretty Tomboy

Cameron Diaz, Kelly Ripa, and Kristen Stewart qualify for this club. If you live in jeans with cute boots or flip-flops and a frilly top, you're in the club, too. Compared to the Contemporary Bohemian or Feminine Frill Seeker, you're more rock-and-roll and bad girl in your sexy style attitude, more Joan Jett than Katie Holmes. You're always looking for ways to dress up a pair of jeans, and you own more pairs of them than you do trousers (and you probably have no skirts). *Sexy stockups for any day:* A fitted biker-style cotton sateen (or leather) jacket; a body-skimming tank or tee with a low-key accent like tonal beading, sequins, or chiffon edges; skinny jeans or pants; and gold hoop earrings.

Remember, the overall point here is to find a place that gets you thinking about who you are, how you want to present yourself, and how to turn your closet into a sexy-style sanctuary, where every choice has a thread of seduction, a neckline just revealing enough, a cut that flatters your assets, or an accessory with a texture that begs to be touched. Sparking up a sexy style can also be as simple as having a sweater in that special color that makes your eyes pop. Just visualizing yourself wearing the perfect things (maybe you're flipping through a catalog over your morning coffee) will get you excited because knowing who you are is a delicious discovery indeed.

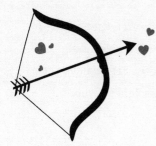

EXERCISE

❤ *Photograph Your Fave Outfits*

Take the guesswork out of that *What can I wear today?* moment by creating a simple photo catalog of your best sexy outfits. You'll glance at it, and before you know it, you'll be dolled up and feeling fabulous. To start, have a try-on night where you style a million looks and narrow them down to a handful of no-fail knockouts. Invite a girlfriend over for support and a second opinion. Lay each ensemble out on your bed or the floor, complete with accessories (shoes, bag, jewelry), and take digital snapshots. Then print a contact sheet with all the looks, and keep it handy so you can consult it and morph *I'm not sure* fashion moments into confident ones—because you'll know when you head out the door that you look irresistible.

LINGERIE YOU LOVE
(AND LOVE YOUR BODY IN)

Besides being a sweet secret under your outfits, well-fitting lingerie can help your clothes look more tantalizing by supporting your breasts and cupping your bottom. When you shop, always slip a shirt on over a bra so you can be certain it sets your bust up to be its most sumptuous, juicy shape.

Before we get into sexy lingerie for seduction, let's talk about everyday underwear. Once you've got your "outer" sexy style rocking, your underthings should get in line, and play an equal (if not greater!) role in igniting your self-confidence. Before you hit the stores to stock up on everyday underwear that rocks your Mojo (because donning humdrum skivvies is a missed opportunity), you're going to want to tap into your lingerie personality to help you choose the sexy underthings that are most representative of you. This quick quiz will help.

WHAT'S YOUR LINGERIE STYLE?

TO DEFINE *your lingerie needs, you're going to need to know your lingerie personality, right? Take the short test below to find out what yours is . . . then, shop accordingly!*

1. My ideal daytime bra is . . .

a) Feminine and soft, with a subtle pattern
b) A clean classic T-shirt bra
c) Sleek and bold, with push-up action
d) Sassy peekaboo style

2. When I want a pattern, I usually buy . . .

a) Lace
b) Something simple, like a contrasting waistband
c) Animal prints, like cheetah
d) No pattern—sheer all the way!

3. I'd love a sexy nightie that's . . .

a) Soft and flowing

b) Like a long T-shirt, but sexier

c) Formfitting with cutout panels or slits

d) I sleep nude, baby!

4. My underwear drawer has . . .

a) Pastel hipsters and bikini bottoms

b) Frilly boy shorts and rump-loving cheeky shorts

c) 100 percent G-strings and thongs

d) Underwear?

5. The sexy costume that's totally me is . . .

a) An angel

b) A sexy football minx

c) A naughty nurse

d) A dominatrix, of course

Now find out how your answers add up

IF YOU CHOSE MOSTLY As . . . YOU'RE A ROMANTIC!

Soft and fluttering, subtly sheer, classic, and comfy shapes and styles . . . these are all your hallmarks when it comes to your lingerie style. Your soft, warm, sweetly romantic nature desires feminine delights that reflect it in kind. Seek out bras with a touchable feel and a softer line to them, like an all-lace bralette for downtime (or if you prefer more support, go for something with an underwire that still has a soft look, like a demi-bra style with scalloped edges), and look for matching panties with equally sumptuous fabrics that give you coverage, but not so much so that you're wearing bloomers!

IF YOU CHOSE MOSTLY Bs . . . YOU'RE SPORTY AND SWEET!

You're fun and playful, and your underthings should be, too. Your lingerie needs should lean to the spunkier side, with pieces that are reflective of your hot tomboy nature (while adding form and function). You like clean styles that are a little edgy and boyish at once, like cottons that stretch and hug your curves in revealing cuts. But there's no reason what you wear can't have an undercurrent of sex appeal. To spice it up, consider the same tomboy styles in sheer fabrics with point d'esprit detailing—these will appeal to your sweet and sporty sides for sure. Or check out string bikini-style bras, which are so feminine and sporty at once. Stylewise, your panties should be a little cheeky! Try mini-boy shorts that have a men's-briefs look but in hot pink or bright racy red.

IF YOU CHOSE MOSTLY Cs . . . YOU'RE A SEXPOT!

Your calling card is a yummy mix of satin, lace, and ruffles, creating an undeniable allure. Go on the hunt for bombshell classics, like push-up bras that have *oomph* (or at least formed cups that give your girls that look-at-me shape). If you're small chested, try a plunge bra. In a sheer-lace combo, the style is sinfully sexy. Bottoms that fall in the G-string to thong range and have seductive details (like lace-ups in the back or keyholes) are sure to resonate with your bewitching nature. Styles that mix satin, sheer, and lace at once are very you.

IF YOU CHOSE MOSTLY Ds . . . YOU'RE A WILDCAT!

Look out—you're on the prowl! You're an adventurer at heart and love spicy surprises—both giving and receiving—so why not reflect that in your unmentionables? Though you can't always get away with racy peekaboo bras and split-down-the-middle panties, you can certainly pepper your drawer with such goodies for the right moments. Make sure to balance your risqué pieces with functional wear (though functional doesn't have to be boring—there is plenty of decadent "daily" lingerie to choose from at your nearest undies store). Nurture your wild-side look with sheers, lace, and out-there colors or naughty fabrics in a conventional style, like biker-chick fabrics that look like vinyl but are really some sort of breathable silk or cotton.

LINGERIE

BODY BUILDERS

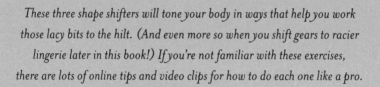

These three shape shifters will tone your body in ways that help you work those lacy bits to the hilt. (And even more so when you shift gears to racier lingerie later in this book!) If you're not familiar with these exercises, there are lots of online tips and video clips for how to do each one like a pro.

💜 **Squats.** Make as though you're sitting back onto a kitchen chair, and with your hands clasped in front for balance, hold the pose midair. That low crouch will burn, but the payoff is seriously hotter buns.

💜 **Planks.** This push-up-like pose targets deep-set abdominal muscles, and that's why doing planks can suck in your stomach, flatten your lower abs, and whittle your waist like no type of crunch. It's the ultimate core-tightening move, meaning it strengthens the entire torso, and it even improves your posture, so you'll stand up straighter, with greater "presence," the way a dancer does.

💜 **Push-ups.** Yep, they're a pain—but they have so many benefits. They work not only your arms and shoulders—giving you a sexy canvas to slide that cami or bra onto—but they also exercise your pectoral muscles, which give your breasts added pop! You can start with the "girl" kind (bent knees) or with wall push-ups. Do three sets of ten, three times a week. However, I want you to always make your first push-up a full-body one because from one, it's not hard to add another, then build up to six, seven, eight! Results will show way faster if full-style push-ups are in your repertoire.

MOJO MOMENT

The feeling of achy muscles the next day actually made me horny. It reminded me of how hard I'd worked my body, and that was a turn-on. It actually moved me to have a fun solo!

—*Colleen, Late Bloomer*

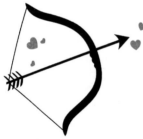

EXERCISE

Find Confidence in the *Lingerie* Department

I want you to immerse yourself in shopping for lingerie as deeply and passionately as you can. Finger the decadent satins and lace, and tune into what you would do to yourself in them or how your partner will become excited seeing you in them. Tickle your skin with satin ribbons and lacy ruffles and imagine them grazing a lover's bare body.

Then, in the fitting room, as you're looking at your bod in that bra, cami, or bikini bottom, I want you to use this opportunity to tell yourself how fabulous you look in it. Remember the exercise where you learned how to turn your negative body banter upside down? Think of this as another seductive body ritual! This is where you can really practice radical self-acceptance and total body love. Your body is gorgeous. It's *yours*, so own it!

Last, remember this is about you—choose pieces to buy because *you* love them. Although it's great to snap

up goodies that entice and make your lover hunger for you, your partner will want you even more when your confidence is sky-high, courtesy of that bralette you just *love* to wear. Captivate *yourself* first, and the rest will fall deliciously into place!

I hope you're starting to discover and embrace your sexy style and lingerie personality. Wearing lingerie has become one of my greatest joys. Call me vain; call me silly, but pulling on silky, sexy, and comfortable lingerie and checking myself out in the mirror makes me totally alluring. Of course lingerie can add heat to your relationship, but whether you're single or coupled up, wearing ever-so-sexy underthings is one of the easiest ways to boost your Mojo on a daily basis. And once you get it, you'll see your basic underwear drawer transform into a prized possession, a treasure trove you hit up every morning to give you a little daily seduction in your step.

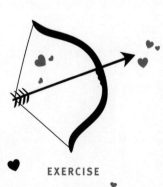

EXERCISE

Strut Your Stuff!

I'm sure you're on top of the world with your newfound sexy style and that you're dying to get it out there. In fact, it's a must for this week. Work it in public! Drink up the reactions you get from others; check yourself out in every mirror or store window you pass by and enjoy the boost! As soon as you get home, I want you to jot down in your journal how you felt before, during, and after your outing. Congrats on a job well done!

LET'S KEEP THE SEXY NEW EXPERIENCES COMING.
NEXT UP, YOU'LL LEARN HOW EASY IT CAN BE
TO TURN YOUR BEDROOM INTO A
SANCTUARY OF SEDUCTION. GET READY
TO DIM THOSE BRIGHT OVERHEAD LIGHTS AND SEE
HOW MOJO MAGICAL YOUR BOUDOIR CAN BE.

CHAPTER NINE

Make Over Your Bedroom

Y OU'VE BEEN WORKING HARD TO INFUSE EVERY POSSIBLE MOMENT and experience in your world with a little bit of sex appeal—and now, we're taking it into the bedroom! Say good-bye to unsexy clutter and hello to an environment that really lights your fire. After all, you'll be having a lot of action in this space. So it makes sense that it should be a place that turns you on and makes you feel seductive and free to experiment (with yourself and others)! And as you've learned, the more action you're having, the sexier your energy will be and the more you'll be attracting others into your life and into your bed.

Now it's time to learn the steps that will transform your bedroom into an oasis for seduction. You're going to clean things up (literally) and tweak the decor so it exudes more *ooh la la*.

Get ready—you're about to transform your bedroom into a frolic-friendly playground.

WHAT'S YOUR BEDROOM STYLE?

Much like a killer outfit, your bedroom shouldn't be a clash of styles. At this point, you've already had to think about some broad-stroke style preferences. The same clues for a wardrobe generally carry over to how you like your personal space to look. These prompts can help you translate those clues into the decor arena, so you can start your to-do list.

Style type: Feminine Frill Seekers

YOU'LL LIKE: ROMANTIC LOOKS. Think flowers; candles; shabby chic–style chandeliers; and muted colors like chocolate, mocha, or pinks (or for a romantic cottage feel, light blues, white, and light neutrals and white molding and beadboard). You'd love a feminine upholstered headboard inspired by Marie Antoinette, but suitable for today—call it Antoinette light!—in a floral or lush velvet. Cottage lovers likely prefer beds that lend themselves to being wrapped with gauzy, sheer curtains that can billow in the breeze. A dressing table is a romantic must, with a silver tray to hold decorative perfume bottles or an antique silver-handled brush-and-comb set.

Style type: Modern Minimalists + Pretty Tomboys

YOU'LL LIKE: CONTEMPORARY AND MODERN. An overall clean style with little wall decoration is your ideal. You prefer that a modern headboard, a graphically designed chaise lounge, or a cool rug double as pieces of art and serve as focal points. Interesting fabric is more important to you than intricate styling or details. The same goes for furniture and lamps—you gravitate toward smooth lines rather than ornate carved looks. For a color scheme, neutrals—

like grays, beiges, and whites—in varying complementary tones add depth and interest. If you're looking to buy a new bed at any point soon, consider a low platform bed. (Tip: muted, tonal bedding that's in the same family as your carpet or flooring can make your current frame appear lower because the bed will blend into the floor.) A lamp splurge would be minimalistic paper lamps that can be set to softly illuminate the room.

Style type: Contemporary Bohemians

YOU'LL LIKE: BORDELLO CHIC. No doubt, it will appeal to your vintage sensibilities. Imagine a 1920s speakeasy, with a dark, plush look. Boas, lace, draped or layered fabrics; saturated jewel-tone colors, like ruby red (a chaise in a dark-on-dark toile); mysterious lighting, like wall sconces that cast low accent light only. You may love wrought-iron accessories on the wall for a darker, sexy, even gothic feel. Hints of animal print, mirrors, funky lamps appeal to you. So do flowing satin drapes and table coverings—a bedside table covered with tasseled, beaded fabric and topped with glass. An exotic-looking, far-eastern print rug in jewel tones might be your choice to round out the sinfully sexy energy, but richly plush accent rugs also connote luxe self-indulgence and would feel so satisfying under your naked feet, or on your back!

EASY WAYS TO ADD MOJO
TO YOUR BOUDOIR

If you're adding new decorative items, think ahead: pull inspirational photos from magazines and catalogs to create a visual game plan and shopping list.

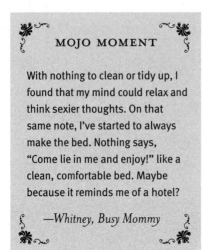

MOJO MOMENT

With nothing to clean or tidy up, I found that my mind could relax and think sexier thoughts. On that same note, I've started to always make the bed. Nothing says, "Come lie in me and enjoy!" like a clean, comfortable bed. Maybe because it reminds me of a hotel?

—*Whitney, Busy Mommy*

Doing so will help you stay in the style you chose from above—everything will work together that way. (Paste some of the inspirational photos onto your Mojo Motivation Board, too!)

Keep in mind that you want to be doing a lot of touching in the bedroom (touching yourself and your lover), and having items you want to caress is great inspiration for that. Search for pillows with textures you want to rub your skin against—perhaps satin, lace, or delicate strips of leather fringe. These simple quick fixes will help give an immediate sass-up to your bedroom.

On a budget? Read on—many of these sexy upgrades require little or no money at all!

♥ **Ditch the clutter.** Your surroundings influence your life and mood. I know that when my home is a cluttered mess, I feel frustrated, claustrophobic, and totally unsexy. File away those tax documents already! Throw the outdated cards away or put them in a special keepsake box in your closet. Move exercise equipment to another room (a treadmill is so unsexy, and if you're using it to hang jeans on, that's even worse!), toss the stacks of old magazines, and sweep away the dust bunnies that have collected behind them.

💜 **Make the space work, kid, in-law free.** Jettison any traces of work; they're a reminder of things you need to do, of a stressful week ahead. Similarly, hide your laptop (unless you plan on watching something sexy on it). Clear out family photos with anyone who shouldn't be watching you have sex—send your mother-in-law to the den. Kids toys are a reminder that you're a great parent, but not a sexy mama! Stow them in their proper place. It's all a distraction from putting your Mojo first.

💜 **Place your furniture thoughtfully.** Do what you can to improve the flow of your space. A clear path will make the room feel more comfortable and welcoming—you'll want to linger more because it won't feel so erratic. There's nothing sexy about knocking your shins against a chair. If there are simply too many pieces of furniture in your room, you've got to thin them out.

MOJO MOMENT

I'm single, and before, I wouldn't have thought about using blatantly sexy bedding. It seemed like something you had when you lived with someone. But duh! I did it for me. It is literally a pleasure to slip into the sheets by myself. I find I reach into my "naughty" bedside drawer much more now.

—*Tessa, Late Bloomer*

♥ **Upgrade your drapes.** Window dressings can definitely enhance your sexy new bedroom. I love gauzy, flowing drapes, because they're a little exhibitionist (though, of course, keep in mind your neighbors and what they can see!). If your bedroom style is richer and more dramatic, decorate your windows with rich heavy drapes that you can draw closed to shut out the world.

♥ **Use light to flatter and seduce.** Lighting creates intimacy and warmth. Be sure you can adjust your lamps and overhead fixtures with dimmers or different settings (like with three-way bulbs, which may very well inspire raunchy three-way thoughts every time you twist the knobs!). Chandeliers dripping in crystals are always sexy. Warm light from candles and light-filtering lampshades or amber-tinted sconce covers add enchantment. Even stringing up some delicate little twinkly lights can add romance and fantasy.

♥ **Seek out pleasurable bedding.** You want soft, luscious, plush, heavenly blankets and sheets against your naked skin. Silks, good satins, high-quality silky cotton, and soft-spun wool (for blankets and throws) feel super sexy. If you're on a budget, I recommend picking up cotton jersey sheets. They're so soft against your naked skin you'll never wear pajamas to bed again!

♥ **Set a sultry mood with fragrance.** Scent can be a big turn-on in your bedroom. It will transport you away from your workday and into your own personal sexy playground instantly. Light candles and burn oils—think vanilla, musk, sandalwood, even a hint of cinnamon, or something with a subtle combination of sweet and spicy.

♥ **Stock a seductive book.** No matter how sexy your bedroom looks, there's always room for a little extra stimulation to get you in the mood. So keep an anthology of sexy stories or a book of provocative photography at your bedside table. You can look at it on your own and fantasize or thumb through it with your lover and discuss what's sexy about each story or photo. It might lead to a sexy journaling—or photo—session of your very own! Need a bookmark? Use a photo of yourself from a time when you felt on fire.

♥ **Keep treats nearby.** Having little bites of chocolate in a delicate glass bowl next to the bed is sexy because chocolate and sex go together and a little bite of dark chocolate heaven is a perfect reward after you've had an incredible orgasm!

I want you to do as many of these suggestions as you can within reason over the next few days. I understand that some larger changes might take time to pull together, but you'll find that simple steps like ridding the clutter will have noticeable impacts right away.

IT'S TIME TO PUT YOUR MOJO WHERE YOUR
MOUTH IS. NEXT UP: YOU'LL LEARN HOW
TO TALK OUT WHAT YOU NEED
FROM YOUR LOVER TO REACH THE BLISS
THAT YOU WANT AND THE PLEASURE YOU DESERVE.
GET READY TO TAKE CHARGE OF YOUR
SEX SATISFACTION!

This Week's Mojo Mission

HAVE THE SEX YOU NEED—AND DESERVE

It's still early in the Mojo Makeover, but that doesn't mean you can't start to cash in on the fruits of your labors! This week the transformation really begins. Start your libidos!

GET READY TO

- ♥ Feel fully at ease talking with your partner about your sexual needs.

- ♥ Have five orgasms as part of the Big 5-O program.

- ♥ Open your mind (and bedroom) up to some lusty accessories.

- ♥ Say things that you never have before . . . and enjoy it.

KEEP UP THE GOOD MOJO WORK!

Update your girlfriends on your progress! Schedule a girls' lunch or have an iChat session with a friend who lives across the country.

CHAPTER TEN

Communicate Your Desires

ALTHOUGH SEX STARTS IN THE MIND, IT MATURES, DEVELOPS, and evolves through communication. To cultivate a fully frisky and enviable Mojo, you've got to talk about sex! Good sexual communication will help you create the spicy life you want *and* deserve, but sometimes it's hard to find the words—and then figure out how to use them.

First, know that nerves are normal—and that applies to anyone, whether you've been with a partner for two months, two years, or twelve years. Even someone who's well versed in disclosing his or her deepest desires gets tongue-tied from time to time. But take a deep breath, have some patience with yourself, and soon you'll be verbal in ways that you never dreamed.

If you're with a partner and you haven't been engaging in regular, open, and loving sex communication with him, starting to talk about it now may feel a little awkward at first. But it's important in so many ways. It's more than about creating just the sex life that you want with your partner—it's also about creating that intimate connection that allows both of you to have openness in other areas of your relationship, too. The ability to have deep discussions about your more primal and loving moments helps you both to build trust . . . and the more trust you build, the deeper you can go with your sexual explorations!

If you're not with a partner yet, these lessons still apply to you. (Sometimes, the partner you need to communicate your desires to is actually . . . you!) Don't let your fabulous singlehood stand in the way of learning good sexy-talk skills that you can put into use later in this book when we get down and dirty with dirty talk.

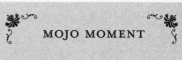

MOJO MOMENT

I told my guy that I'd like to try having synchronized orgasms. I explained that during sex I have one or two smaller orgasms but that I'd really like to work on building to the climax together. He told me that part of the problem may be that sometimes he focuses on getting me to orgasm first so that he feels he's done a good job, then he'll orgasm afterward. I told him that I'd rather him not worry so much about my O but try to tune in to our energy together and ride the wave to the climax together. He said he'd like to try that, too. Yes!!!

—*Naomi, Frustrated Fox*

Okay, let's get that mind of yours churning out some salacious thoughts!

OPENING UP THE LINES OF COMMUNICATION WITH YOUR LOVER

When it comes to talking about sex with an intimate partner, the most common concern I hear is, *How do I start?* We'll get into more advanced communication approaches in later chapters with lessons on fun and frisky dirty talk, but for now, here's a basic framework to kick off your conversations.

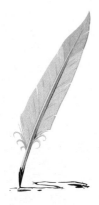

**JOURNALING
EXERCISE**

Sex-Life Satisfaction—
Time to Check In

First, use your journal to write about what's really working in your sex life right now and what you'd like to change up.

WHAT'S GREAT. Are you satisfied with the frequency of your sexual activity? The playfulness or intimacy of your encounters? The intensity of your orgasms? What else?

WHAT COULD BE BETTER. Are your sex drives out of sync? Do you wish that your lover would initiate more so that you feel wanted? Are you stuck in a routine or having trouble reaching orgasm? What else?

Now, how do you translate these thoughts into a loving discussion? First, you need to choose the right time and place to have the conversation—and let me tell you one thing I know for sure; that right time and place is not naked in the bedroom, before, during, or immediately after sex. It's too vulnerable a space for you and your mate. Instead, bring it up when you're both relaxed, perhaps when you're out to dinner or in front of the fireplace and you're sharing some wine. As you're about to broach the subject, find ways to feel physically close to your lover—touch him and allow for time to get comfortable with each other. Remember, this isn't a board meeting or a contract negotiation!

Approach the conversation with love and tenderness. Try not to interrupt. Ask questions. Many people are hesitant to reveal their deepest thoughts out of fear of rejection or ridicule. So be patient, and remember to listen so your partner feels free to be part of the discussion. And most of all, let respect guide you.

Discussion dos

To get things started, try an opener like, "Babe, I'd love to talk a little about our sex life. Can I share something with you?" Then, your next sentence should lead with a positive affirmation, like, "I love the way we _____, and I want us to take it to a whole other level." (Your list from the journaling exercise above can help here.) It's good to focus on the positive so that both you and your partner acknowledge that there are things that are working, and so that he doesn't feel you're in "attack" mode.

Or you might say: "I love the way we've always been so affectionate in public, it makes me feels sexy and connected to you, and I'd love to bring that intimacy into the bedroom by _____." Have a sexy suggestion ready to fill in the blank, like that you want to pick up some new lingerie or a sexy toy for you both or tell him about a few new positions you've read about.

It's easier to navigate a sticky conversation like this (especially with an insecure partner or a new one) by offering up some ideas, and frankly, most partners will feel turned on that you did some sexy research ahead of time. Sharing some book passages or sexy magazine articles would be one idea. Ask for your lover's input. It will help your partner feel more connected to the experience and more invested in wanting to help you create the sex life you ultimately desire. And that's a good place to be!

More suggestions

- ♥ I would love more hugs and *I love you*s outside the bedroom and throughout the day, and to kiss and snuggle more when we're in bed; it makes me feel close to you.

- ♥ I'd love for us to have a sexual marathon. Let's lock ourselves into the bedroom for an afternoon and explore each other's body and touch and tease and see what kind of Os we can uncover that way.

❤ I would love to try some new things with you, like some new positions—maybe some fantasy role-playing or incorporating some fun props, like a cool new vibrator or satin handcuffs, into our playtime.

Discussion don'ts

Whatever you do, *don't* say,

❤ I'm really enjoying the sex we're having, but I feel that there are some areas I'd like to improve in.

❤ I'm still really sexually attracted to you, but I've been having trouble reaching orgasm lately, and I'd like to work on that together.

❤ I enjoy our lovemaking sessions so much, but I'd really like to explore some new experiences that could be a lot of fun for both of us.

They're honest, yes; however, they're laced with criticism, and the last thing you want is to make your lover feel insecure. Avoid turning your phrases with a *but*. As in, this works, *but* . . . It negates the kind words that come before it. Better: suggest a positive solution so you end on an upswing.

As a final step to this exercise, I invite you to encourage your lover to share in the same way with you. Ask him the same questions—What does he need? What does he desire? What does he want from you? This will help you hear feedback of the same nature from his perspective, and give you the opportunity to help fulfill his hungers.

REMEMBERING
THE BASICS OF SEX TALK

As you continue to work with the scripts above to help you to deliver your deepest desires to your partner in a constructive way, your formula for discussion will stay the same, but the words, phrasing, and approach will evolve. Even so, there are some constants you definitely want to bear in mind!

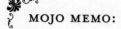

MOJO MEMO:

Speak Before You Speak

Before you venture into this confessional communication with your lover, take some time out to gather your thoughts, and practice saying them out loud in front of a mirror. Unless it's already a comfortable topic of conversation between you and your mate, this is not a subject you want to speak impulsively on.

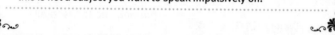

♥ **Keep it positive.** There will be times when—despite your best attempts at talking over what you want—your partner may not deliver what you hoped for. Maybe he's overly attentive to one part or using a tad too much friction on another. It's going to be tempting to tell him what's not working, but stop yourself before those words leave your lips. Instead of saying what's not right, point him in a new direction. Sex is a vulnerable time for both of you, and being shot down (however gently) is a definite Mojo buster. An easy way to transition him from one not-awesome move into a yummier one is to touch *him* in a specific way and then invite him to do the same to you. Or more directly, take his fingers in yours and show him what titillates you. Be sure to *purr* in his ear that it feels good.

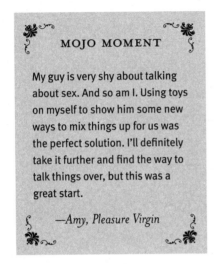

MOJO MOMENT

My guy is very shy about talking about sex. And so am I. Using toys on myself to show him some new ways to mix things up for us was the perfect solution. I'll definitely take it further and find the way to talk things over, but this was a great start.

—*Amy, Pleasure Virgin*

♥ **Funny is fabulous.** In the beginning, you're apt to have a few clunkers when you try to step up your sex moves and it doesn't go smoothly. (Maybe you're both just not as bendy as you thought.) And you might laugh, and so will your partner, and that's totally okay. Laughter is a great way to connect, and it tempers any insecurity that might bubble up. It's often in those intimate moments in bed when you feel deliciously close that you'll end up spilling what you're thinking without holding back. Just remember laughter in bed is fine. But talking about how funny it was that he couldn't lift you against the wall is something to do over breakfast, not in the moment.

♥ **Showing racier play makes it easier to discuss later.** It's easier to communicate provocative new desires by first dabbling in the act and following up on them with a conversation. For example, you might try using a fingertip vibrator for some light anal-spot play on yourself while he watches, or try it on *his* A-Spot. During the hot moment, share how you feel about the sexy sensations with a randy cry-out. Or as he writhes and moans, comment that you can tell he likes it, and say that you would like to try it, too.

♥ **Be patient with a nonchatty lover.** You might think that by revealing what excites you, your lover will do the same, but it's not always the case. If yours isn't free with words, don't push too hard. Instead, coax it out by including him as a key player when you explain what you want. If he sees your explorations include him, he'll feel more confident.

♥ **You can't compliment too much or too often.** I constantly hear stories from women who compliment their lovers' technique inside the bedroom or compliment it outside the bedroom. Why not do both? Some *I love how you do that*'s and *Please don't stop*'s and *That feels amazing*'s go a long way toward getting you what you want out of your bedroom experience, but dropping those tasty little tidbits into out-of-bedroom conversations tells him that you're still riding high on the memory of the experience. And on top of that, it gets you both turned on and thinking about doing what you loved all over again!

The more you work on you sexual communication, and continue to think about sex in new and exciting ways, the firmer your foundation becomes in building a lasting, desirable sex life. And the best part? You also create a deeper, more intimate connection to your own Mojo.

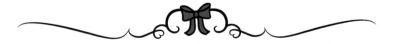

NO DOUBT YOU'VE GOTTEN YOURSELF
ALL WORKED UP WITH ALL OF THIS SEXY THINKING
AND TALKING! I HOPE IT WILL INSPIRE YOU
IN THE NEXT CHAPTER. ARE YOU READY TO FOCUS
ON YOUR GORGEOUS PLEASURE FOR A WHILE?
LET'S GO!

CHAPTER ELEVEN

The Big 5-O Program

N O QUESTION, AN ORGASM LEAVES YOU FLOATING ON A CLOUD
of tingling electric happiness and makes you feel amazing,
courtesy of a pure moment of selfish pleasure and indulgence. So
it's time to have more! Taking part in the Big 5-O program means
devoting yourself to having five orgasms a week. They can be long-
drawn-out sessions or quickies, done solo or with a partner, or any
combo of your choosing.

Where did I come up with five? It's a doable amount. (I swear. It
is!) It's frequent enough to encourage you to explore different roads
to your pleasure, and I know that after a week you'll be pleasantly
surprised by how it isn't a huge hurdle at all. Five will inspire (and
require!) you to get creative, and that in turn will give you a broader
view of what an O can be. Also, the more Os you have, the easier
and faster they'll happen for you, and the more you'll want. Having
more orgasms will further infuse your life with sexiness, build a

stronger connection to and acceptance of your body, and encourage more goodness to come your way! You'll find yourself invigorated and inwardly proud of your 5-O accomplishment. When you're out and about, you'll have a new glow—everyone you see will notice that there's suddenly something electric about you!

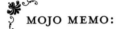

MOJO MEMO:

Explaining the Why of Os

I'll never forget the day my mom talked to me about masturbation. I was thirteen or fourteen, and she said, "Sex with someone you love will be great, and I'd prefer if you waited until you were older. But did you know that treating yourself to sexual pleasure could be just as good? Masturbation is totally normal and healthy."

I quickly ran out of the room to avoid any further details, but what she effectively did for me, in just two sentences, was give me the okay to do something I already felt was quite natural. I was already in tune with sexual feelings and sensations and had begun exploring sexy solo sessions, but it was her approval that removed any shame. Nicely done, Mom! Her open communication about the topic allowed me to grant myself the permission to have a healthy, satisfying relationship with myself.

Through practice and frequency, I got to know myself sexually but also emotionally. Learning about my body this way gave me an added layer of self-knowledge and self-acceptance that helped me feel like a more complete person.

This is why I'm so passionate about the Big 5-O program. It will help you connect the dots and take in the *whole* you. It'll remind you that you're not just a mother or a professional or the best in your boot-camp class. You've got this rich inner life . . . an inner vixen that you know better than anyone else, and she's a source of power, joy, confidence, and pure femininity.

For those who've never had a sexy solo session: Be patient. It may take you a couple tries to let yourself go and reach the Big O. Or, it may just take a minute, and you'll laugh with pleasure and then perhaps burst into tears because you'll wonder what kept you from this kind of connection with yourself for so long.

But, to all of you ladies—give yourself permission to go for it, to commit to this, to go for the glow!

DID YOU KNOW...
Os ARE GOOD FOR YOU?

There are a lot of reasons to have more Os. Of course they feel beyond amazing! But they have health and vitality benefits that you might not be aware of, and they play a role in maximizing your sexy self-confidence to boot! Here's a quick look at the reasons to fit more Os into your life.

♥ Studies suggest sex helps people live longer by releasing antibodies that boost the immune system. (Fewer pesky head colds!)

♥ The release of a hormone oxytocin, also called the "love hormone," appears to encourage bonding, trust, and love. We could all use more of that!

♥ Your body is flooded with endorphins after orgasm—they're the same chemicals released after exercise—making you feel euphoric, calm, and centered. It's hard to be in a bad mood after one!

♥ Because they're de-stressers, Os help you sleep better.

♥ The more orgasms you have, the better you'll get to know your body and what it likes. In other words, you'll develop pleasure skills, and that's empowering!

♥ All these benefits promote better self-esteem. How so? The better you feel physically and mentally (including logging in better sleep time), the happier you'll be.

THE SWEET PATHS TO O−LATION

You probably know the basic type of Os. But in brushing up on the wheres and hows, I find there's always a tidbit of *who knew!* to pick up on, and that can help spark creativity and lead to better, bigger, more. Check out these three types of orgasms and think about whether you're getting what you *O* so deserve in your sex life.

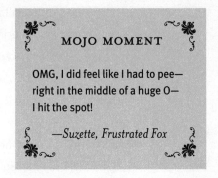

- **C-Spot.** For starters, there's the clitoral orgasm. This type is reached through direct stimulation of the clitoris, which is the fleshy knob located just north of your vaginal opening. The clitoris is much like a penis in that during arousal it becomes engorged thanks to increased blood flow, and with this, it becomes more and more sensitive to the touch. Your lady petals (the soft, sensitive folds that cover your C- and V-Spots till you part them) also become engorged and sensitive to pleasurable sensations, and you'll find that light stroking or oral stimulation during foreplay is a tantalizing treat. Try it to create a slow burn that makes C-Spot pleasure even more explosive.

> **MOJO MOMENT**
>
> OMG, I did feel like I had to pee—right in the middle of a huge O—I hit the spot!
>
> —*Suzette, Frustrated Fox*

- **G-Spot.** A G-Spot orgasm happens inside the vagina. The G-Spot is thought to be a small spongy orb that's chock-full of nerve endings. Some experts believe it's actually an extension of the C-Spot, and that its nerve pathways can be stimulated from the inner V-wall. To stimulate your G-Spot, insert a finger (with your

palm up toward your belly button) and make a come-hither motion with that finger against the front wall of your vagina. (Most women will say they feel as though they have to pee when it's being stimulated—but don't worry; you won't!) There are also vibrators with curved arms specifically made to stroke the G-Spot. These tools are quite helpful because G-Spot Os aren't as easy to come by as C-Spot ones, but they're worth practicing because they're intense. Dedicate yourself to G exploration and see what bubbles up!

💜 **Blended Os.** This is the holy grail of Os. It's when your C-Spot and G-Spot are simultaneously stimulated and create a deep, earth-shaking, intense orgasm (more intense than when you have a C- or G-Spot orgasm on its own). Some toys—like rabbit-style vibrators—target both spots at once for a doubly hot sensation of internal and external stimulation.

YOUR 5-O MISSION

So once again, your goal is to have five orgasms over the course of seven days. You can have them with a toy, a boy, your favorite boy toy. Go for it in the tub, in traffic, wherever you can make it happen! (Feel free to bang out two of your weekly five in one session if you like.) During your mission, I want you to keep track of your O satisfaction in your journal (check out the samples on page 143).

Remember, the point of the 5-O program is to explore. There are *unlimited* scenarios that you can discover solo or with a partner. Whether you're in a

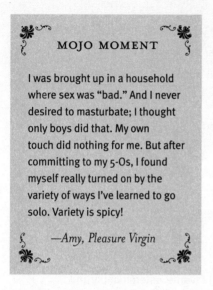

relationship or satisfying yourself, I encourage you to spice things up with new toys and wild positions.

As part of the 5-O program, I want you to think *variety*. We all have that one go-to toy, position, or pressure point that we love because it gets us there every time, and that's fabulous— use it! It's great if a special vibrator can get there in thirty-five seconds, but what if you worked against a pillow or blanket? Or used two toys at once? (It will create the aura of two partners at once—hot!) Or if oral sex is what normally gets you off, add a toy into the session for a new sensation. You can even include your partner directly—a couples toy that stimulates you both during intercourse is another treat to try; it can bring you there together.

READY, SET, O!

At the end of the day, no two Os are alike, and no matter how orgasmic you already are, there is a whole world of self-discovery out there. Solo sessions are all about you and discovering more about yourself and the sexual creature that you are. If you find yourself faking it with a partner because you can't get there or don't feel you can communicate what you need to blast off, solo sessions will help you learn what you love, and you can teach that to a lover. So go ahead and pleasure yourself right in front of your lover and don't feel shy at all. Trust me, your partner wants you to have that O, and watching you make it happen will be a huge turn-on.

Self-service

Need inspiration for solo sessions? Here are some of my favorite moments for grabbing a quick O. They send me to the strat-O-sphere every time! Try 'em or tweak 'em into something that becomes your own hot moment.

- ♥ **A.M. quickie.** This is a simple shower booster to try as you get ready for the morning—grab your favorite waterproof toy and charge yourself up! It's the perfect way to start the day on an invigorated sexy note.

- ♥ **Lunchtime stress reliever.** There are many incognito toys you can pack in your bag to use at the office on a lunch break. Booty Parlor's LipTrick looks like a lipstick, and the TouchUp is a dead ringer for a bottle of nail polish—no one will know the difference! Getting busy in your brain will minimize how much time you spend in the stall, which might matter if it's a shared office bathroom and a line is forming outside the door. Fantasize a sexy scenario for five minutes so you're mentally turned on before you head to the staff ladies' room. Use the time to *anticipate* that gorgeous O! If you're at home, you can use the same warm-up technique and then sneak off while the baby's sleeping or grab some fast alone time before the kids get home from school.

❤ **Workout warm-up.** I like to have a quick one before I head to the gym because it gets me in tune with my body, and then I'm more connected to my physical fitness. It puts me in a better workout mood, too. Sometimes I do it after because I get turned on looking in the mirror as I dance, sculpt, and sweat—my body's strength and endurance is hot!

❤ **Traffic time waster.** I live in Los Angeles, where waiting in fully stopped traffic is a normal part of daily life. I sometimes pass the time with a pocket vibrator. It makes me have less road rage! This isn't for everyone; you need to have a car where you ride high up (like an SUV) and good control over your facial expression so others don't see you (if you don't care if others see your O face, good for you!). Just make sure that your car is at a full stop!

❤ **Stress fix.** Maybe there's a problem at the office or my husband and I got into a snarky tiff or PMS is pushing my mood to witchy places where everything ticks me off. After indulging in a stress-fixing O, I'm always gifted with a sense of having a blank slate; the stress is dialed down, and I can reboot my brain and steer the rest of the day or night the way I want it to be.

♥   **Date with yourself.** This is for when you've set aside the time to create a seductive oasis with candles, toys, and sexy music. A sumptuous bubble bath would be spot-on (so to speak!). It's important to have these moments because they're chances to work your way up slowly, using different strokes, speeds, and pressure, from delicate to quick. Use these dates to perfect the art of bringing yourself to the brink and dialing it back, then back up to an even more explosive O than ever before!

REACHING YOUR O WITH A PARTNER

These positions and props will help you discover new ways to climax when you're getting frisky with a lover.

♥   **Take the top spot.** It's easier for a woman to orgasm against a partner if she's on top and her partner is lying back (or he can be sitting up, as long as she's on top). It puts you in control of the friction, rhythm, and position of your C-Spot against your mate's body.

♥   **Choose a position that allows your partner clear access to your C-Spot while he's in you.** You can also throw a toy into the mix for a truly wild ride.

♥   **Lube up.** The slippery sensation of personal lubricant mimics your natural slip, and it makes gliding a finger around easier,

Warm Yourself up for a Hot Solo O

Ideally, you've been seeking out sexiness in little things as you go

about your day (your own image in the mirror, seductively shaped

bottles in a gourmet store, or a ten-second fantasy about a hot guy

at your gym . . . or your kid's peewee-league coach). Thinking

saucy thoughts all day will have you red-hot for yourself or

your bedmate.

which is: (1.) a turn-on for your partner that invites exploration,
and (2.) makes your partner's touch more sensational—by
reducing friction. Caresses become deliciously butterfly-like. (It'll
help your handiwork on him, too.)

♥ **Sweet treats invite oral exploration.** Your partner won't be able to
resist tasting a chocolate body drizzle or honey or whatever you
whip up.

♥ **Get flat on *your* back.** Your partner will better be able to easily
rub his shaft or fingers against your G-Spot in this position. Tilt
your pelvis up slightly to help him make good contact against
you, or prop your rump up on a pillow.

- 💜 **Try rear entry.** When you're on all fours, he can penetrate deeply by entering you from behind. You or he can free up a hand to touch your C-Spot while he's bonking you. You may find that the cervical stimulation ignites a new kind of pleasure.

- 💜 **Get a tighter grip.** Remember those Kegel exercises from Chapter 6 (page 80)? Use your sex muscles and *squeeze* on his shaft during intercourse. The close contact can help stimulate a G-Spot orgasm. Try it—you'll never skip your exercises after one!

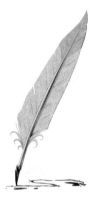

**JOURNALING
EXERCISE**

Keeping an Orgasm Journal

Starting now, and continuing for the rest of your makeover, you're going to journal about every O you have in the 5-O program. Include where you did it, what your inspiration was, what kind of orgasm it was, and how you felt afterward. Go into deep explanation or just keep it really simple with a notation of date, situation, and intensity level . . . but either way it's mandatory. Why? Because having to write about them will help you do them in the first place, and the journal will become a record that shows progression, which is fun and encouraging. During the makeover, you can flip back to be reminded of how great orgasms feel, and to use as erotic reading when you want a lusty boost!

If you're apprehensive about journaling your sexy scenarios, I want you to push yourself. If you can get past your inhibitions, you'll see how it deepens your connection to your Mojo. It will make you feel sexy and powerful and in control, and that in turn will make it comfortable. Of course preventing someone from finding your notes is a simple matter of storing your journal in that perfect hiding spot, and I know you have one. Don't we all, ladies?

Not sure how to get started? Here are a few of my own journal entries to inspire you. Check 'em out!

Sunday night

Had great sex with C. today. A perfect, raw, gorgeous Sunday afternoon session. I had an orgasm through oral sex—no vibrator! So nice. He ran to the grocery afterward, but I was still feeling frisky. So I went for a second O with my fave toy while he was picking up the ingredients for dinner. I kept that second O as my little sexy secret for the evening!

Tuesday afternoon

Feels like I'm getting a cold today. I'm in a bad mood. Want to stay home and relax but I have to drive to the office, ugh . . . But not first without following the 5-O program. If I'm going to preach it, I better practice it! So for inspiration, I surfed for some sexy online clips, and they got my Mojo moving. Just had a great orgasm and am already in a much better mood now. I love that it works every time!

Wednesday

Tonight, I watched Dancing with the Stars *and got turned on by a rather steamy tango—the male*

GOT MULTIPLES?

Multiple orgasms are often thought of as the gold-medal goal that we women should strive for. An actual multiple is when a series of orgasms occur within a short period of time. As soon as one orgasm starts to fade, you continue stimulating and your body then has another and another—they roll into one another. Having more than one O in a session isn't exactly the same thing, but achieving that is super satisfying, too. If you usually call it quits after one, aim for two or three. It's a great way to train your body for multiples. Women need to chill out before they can go again, just as men do. Just rest, so you can reset. Keep a sexy book in your bedside table and read for a few minutes. Or use the time to switch toys for a different mood. Or use a toy meant to revive the fire, like Booty Parlor's The Great Kisser. It's a delicate suction pump that rests over your C-Spot, and when you squeeze it, it draws blood to the spot and ratchets up sensitivity. Doing your Kegels helps, too. Since they strengthen the muscles you use to climax, you'll have more Os.

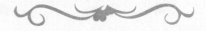

dancer was smoking hot and steaming it up all over the dance floor. Looks like I just stumbled onto today's visual stimulation! I got busy with other things . . . laundry, dinner, e-mails, and such but returned to my mission to have an orgasm. I ran a hot shower, grabbed a waterproof toy, and jumped in for five minutes of bliss. So quick, so easy, and now I'm so relaxed for bed. Tomorrow? I'm making time for another session with the hubs.

And for even more inspiration, here are a few Mojo Model journal entries!

MONDAY

I've been feeling super sexy and ready to start my 5-O program, so I thought I'd bring a mirror and some porn into the mix to kick it off in an extra bold way. I've never had the best self-image, but it started to improve quickly with my Mojo Makeover exercises, and I wanted to see what my boyfriend saw when we were naked. I no longer wanted to be afraid of what I looked liked with the lights on, so I positioned the mirror by my bed, checked out a sexy clip, and went to town with my toys. I actually liked what I saw, and now I truly believe that he likes what he sees, as well. What an amazing start to my 5-O program!

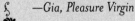
—*Gia, Pleasure Virgin*

THURSDAY

After a long, long day with the kids, I went off for a hot bath with my book. Once in the tub, though, it occurred to me that this was a prime opportunity to work the program. My husband was in the connecting bedroom playing his video games, and his presence added this extra element of urgency to my solo seduction—because I was running the risk of him catching me. It made me feel naughty, hot, and youthful—instead of just exhausted at the day's end!

—*Whitney, Busy Mommy*
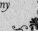

SATURDAY

Tonight I'm going to a friend's engage-ment party. I know for sure a cute boy will be there, so I decide to take extra time to get ready and feel sexy. I put on a soft little slip and pad about the house, feeling super feminine—I'm tuned into my sexiness, so I decide to have a couple Big Os—one with a toy, one without. I put on a sexy black dress and shoes, take time to blow-dry my hair and wear makeup—darker eye shadow than usual. I definitely feel my Mojo all night—in fact, a guy from grad school looks at me halfway through the night and says, "You look hot!"

—*Dara, Late Bloomer*

Hot stuff? Yes, yes, *yes*! Trust me, you're going to discover quickly that orgasms make you more connected to your Mojo. Because of your dedicated O efforts, you'll be experiencing far more satisfaction and will feel more deeply connected to yourself (and your lover if he's in the picture). All of this will, of course, make your sexy self-confidence soar and make others take notice, too. Now enjoy all those Os!

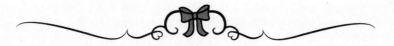

NEXT ON THE MOJO LINEUP . . .
SEXY ACCESSORIES! WHETHER YOU'RE A NOVICE
OR AN OLD PRO AT HAVING FUN WITH THEM,
THIS NEXT CHAPTER IS GOING TO TAKE YOU FOR A
FABULOUSLY FUN, VERY NAUGHTY RIDE. I PROMISE!

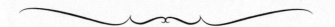

CHAPTER TWELVE

Stock up on Sexy Accessories

HERE'S WHERE WE GET DOWN AND DIRTY WITH SEX TOYS—I'LL run through the options so you can target what gets your motor running. But first, I want to be clear that there are a variety of essential items that *don't* fall under the category of sex toys—let's call these sexy lifestyle accessories. You've experienced a bunch of them already as part of your makeover.

TOOLS THAT ADD SIZZLE
TO YOUR BOUDOIR

Like most areas of a woman's life, we like to accessorize. Think about your beauty routine. Between our makeup and hair accessories, most of us need several drawers to ourselves, if not a separate bathroom to keep our supplies in. For our fitness routines, we have the right shoes, the yoga pants that suit the shape of our bums, the right sports bras to keep the girls feeling good. For work, we have the pens we like, our daily planners, the right rolling briefcases. To me, it's always felt very natural to accessorize my sex life in the same fun feminine way—and to build a collection of sexy accessories that's right in line with my personal preferences.

With Booty Parlor, I've been able to create a whole world of sexy accessories that keep me from having to step into seedy triple-X stores. And even better, I now get to share these new accessory choices with women everywhere—and it's not just about the toys. Instead, there are six core categories of sexy accessories I believe every woman should consider when choosing a collection of tools that suit her sexy lifestyle:

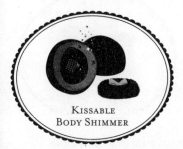

KISSABLE
BODY SHIMMER

1. *Seductive beauty: boost your sexy self-confidence*

These are the primping tools that make you feel sexy the second you use them. They should be part of your daily routine because they make you feel more attractive, more magnetic, more lit up inside. The primping tool can be a plumping lip gloss or a silky shimmering body lotion. It could be that blush that gives you a post-O look, or even a special hair-styling product that leaves your mane looking as if you just rolled around in bed.

2. *Romantic treats: inspire a sexy experience*

Romantic treats are for fun experiential use and can be combined with other sexy toys to create an amazing, intimate sexy experience between lovers. You can

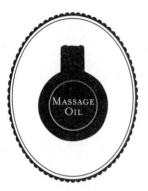

certainly have fun with then on your own, too! Massage oils, lubricants, edible body toppings, massage candles, sexy bubble baths, and enhancement and stimulation gels are also part of this sensual category. So are sweet treats. Why not have a big old spoonful of a rich dark chocolate body fondue after you have a big sexy solo session?

3. Bedroom accessories: try a little frisky business

Bedroom accessories are products that are used to enhance your bedroom play—they are props and tools that create a sexy experience with a partner that goes beyond routine sex and into more exciting, creative sexy experiences. They inspire the exploration of fantasies and add a sense of playfulness to sex. This is where role-playing can come in. Think: bonding tape, whipper ticklers, spankers, wrist cuffs, and blindfolds. By limiting some senses (like blocking out sight or restricting arm movement) you ratchet up others. A feather stroked on your naked skin will feel more succulent

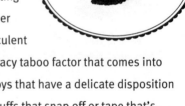

when you're blindfolded. There's definitely a racy taboo factor that comes into play here, and know that there are plenty of toys that have a delicate disposition that keeps things light and fun—like keyless cuffs that snap off or tape that's sticky but easy to remove, no knots needed.

4. Sexy lingerie: play dress up

Flattering lingerie can transform you into a bombshell, a princess, a pinup, or a host of other hot personas. You can be whoever you want, and if you have pieces you love, you'll want to dress up. Keep in mind that pieces you love will be the ones that fit. (There's nothing less sexy than worrying about undies that dig in!) Lingerie that's unique from anything you normally wear will also give an instant lust boost. Booty Parlor's Vibrating

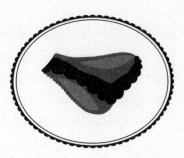

Panties are an example. Having fun with them in public builds anticipation and allows a couple to share a sexy secret together until it's time to ravage each other. It's amazing how undergarments can inspire your inner sexiness!

5. *Love kits: a sexy experience, in a box*

A love kit is a collection of sexy products with a theme that creates a sexy experience. One of the kits I designed has everything you need for a touchy-feely

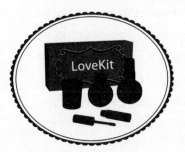

evening (massage oil, lube, body shimmer, and a marabou body feather). Another has a sensually scented candle, sexy peppermint lip gloss, massage oil, and lubricant. Love kits tell a story—about a sexy massage, about a romantic weekend away, or just about pure seduction. They're great to have on hand for a

sexy weekend getaway . . . or just for a sexy solution in a box when you want to create a sexy experience but don't feel like being ultracreative!

6. *Designer sex toys*

Designer sex toys are pleasure objects that address a range of needs and experience levels, from beginner to advanced. The good thing is that sex toys have become very mainstream now, and it's very common for a woman to own one. Why? It's very simple. Vibrators make it easier for women to have orgasms! Your C-Spot loves direct, focused attention and stimulation. Using a toy will definitely quickly enhance and improve your ability to orgasm.

Everything above can certainly be considered a sexy lifestyle accessory, but it doesn't stop there. Your erotic thoughts, journals, books, and videos are sexy tools, as well. Even your new seductively styled bedroom is a sexy tool for your Mojo—it's part of a wide mix of things in your life that can get you worked up! Combining and layering products from the different categories offer you variety and unlimited options to create new sexier experiences that bring you increased satisfaction and pleasure.

Now, let's really explore sex toys! While they're obviously the Shangri-la of sexy accoutrements, you don't want 'em to be the sole means to achieving orgasmic delight. They *can* be star players on your sexual satisfaction team, and for sure, use them to help reach your five Os a week. But because this makeover is about developing a well-rounded sense of sexy self-confidence, I want you to be sure to think of sex toys as the icing on the cake, not the main entrée. Sometimes you should skip them altogether—let your fingers give you joy, too. Mixing things up is the way you'll find out more about yourself and your personal pleasure. Ready to learn what's out there?

SEX TOY ROUNDUP!

Do you *need* to use a sex toy? That's like asking, do you *need* lip gloss? In both cases the answer is no, you don't, but they both make you feel good! Sex toys are tools for fun, for pleasure; they give you something to play with, to get creative with, and ultimately, to get to know yourself better with. A vibrator is a good starting toy, but if another toy sparks desire, by all means, explore it instead!

1. *Vibrators*

Get ready—this is a big category, and each style offers a different experience, so try to bounce around as you build up your collection.

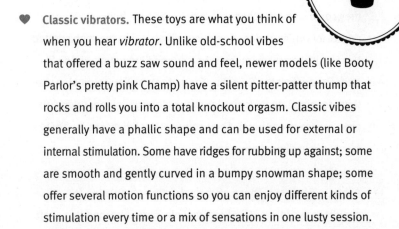

💜 **Classic vibrators.** These toys are what you think of when you hear *vibrator*. Unlike old-school vibes that offered a buzz saw sound and feel, newer models (like Booty Parlor's pretty pink Champ) have a silent pitter-patter thump that rocks and rolls you into a total knockout orgasm. Classic vibes generally have a phallic shape and can be used for external or internal stimulation. Some have ridges for rubbing up against; some are smooth and gently curved in a bumpy snowman shape; some offer several motion functions so you can enjoy different kinds of stimulation every time or a mix of sensations in one lusty session.

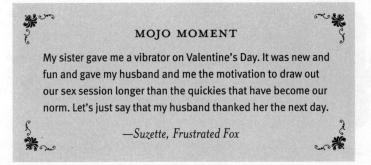

MOJO MOMENT

My sister gave me a vibrator on Valentine's Day. It was new and fun and gave my husband and me the motivation to draw out our sex session longer than the quickies that have become our norm. Let's just say that my husband thanked her the next day.

—*Suzette, Frustrated Fox*

💜 **Sweet and discreet vibes.** These are small toys that offer very targeted sensations and include portable lipstick vibrators and remote-controlled vibrating bullets. A fingertip vibrator is worn on—you guessed it—a finger (it's great for you alone or to use on a partner). Pocket rockets are part of the small and mighty club, too. 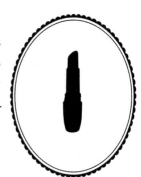 They're the size of small cigars and have vibrating tops. Often they come with interchangeable textured tips, from smooth to ridged, for yummy variety. Contoured vibrators (like the sophisticated Nea) look like art sculptures; their cupped ergonomic shape fits perfectly against the C-Spot . . . and of course you could also use them to stimulate your nipples, trace along your inner thighs, or even arouse your A-Spot. Their compact design makes it easy to maneuver in almost any position.

💜 **Rabbit-style vibes.** These offer dual-action stimulation for simultaneous internal and external pleasure. Attached to a shaft 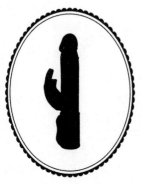 is what looks like a small bunny, and its two rabbit ears are positioned to pitter-patter against your C-Spot while the main shaft stimulates your V-Spot. Besides rabbits, there are versions with dolphins, beavers, and all other sorts of playful animals. There are types with extra bells and whistles, like ones with shafts that gyrate; ones that stimulate with rotating, massaging beads; and even some models that actually thrust up and down. It's easy to understand how Charlotte York became obsessed with a rabbit on *Sex and the City*!

💜 **G-Spot vibes.** These are like classic vibrators but they have curved tips or completely curved bodies. That curve helps find and finesse your G-Spot to bring about intense pleasure. Some G-Spot toys (like Booty Parlor's C-Spot–G-Spot hybrid, Daniel) have additional bumps to help you achieve the coveted blended orgasm.

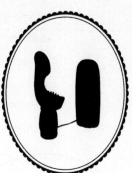

💜 **Wearable vibes.** This is a very unique type of toy that's worn much like a sexy pair of panties. A vibrating butterfly (or heart or

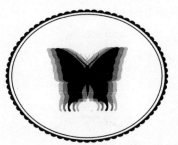

whatever the main vibrator design is) nestles against your lady parts, and the vibrations give incredible direct stimulation. (The butterfly has wings that flutter against your bits to ratchet up the rapture.) Because these vibrators are hands free, you can enjoy their pleasure *while* you're having intercourse, giving oral sex, or on your own vacuuming the house!

💜 **Unique vibes.** There is a growing market of unique wow-factor toys available for you to explore—let's just say they're things that make you go *hmm!* Here are just two of my favorites to consider!

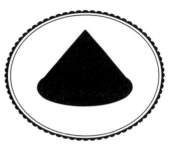

The Cone. What makes this so frisky is the abstract shape. The cone is a pink vibrating silicone pyramid with sixteen different motion patterns. You can straddle it or use it up against a wall or with a partner during intercourse. Because it's unlike most vibrators, I'd recommend it for women who already have vibe experience and want to graduate to something new.

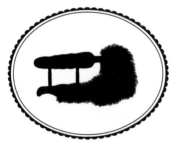

The Minx by Shiri Zinn. This is what I call the Rolls-Royce of sex toys, for those of you who adore luxury (and who doesn't?). The Minx has a luxurious (and generously sized) pink acrylic shaft, a silver base encrusted with twelve pink Swarovski crystals, and a fluffy, pink fully detachable marabou tail. Who says you can't cuddle with a sex toy?

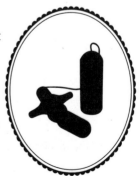

♥ **A-Spot toys.** A-Spot stimulation can be a very exciting part of your sex life—because it feels as though you're exploring something forbidden and racy and because the stimulation can feel amazing and heighten your orgasm like crazy. You can start off with a nonvibrating silicone A-Spot plug or a small vibrating toy designed for A-Spot play (it should have a T-bar or flared base to make sure you don't wind up . . . losing something). There are also A-Spot toys that allow you to experience the fantasy of double penetration—picture a double-ended U-shaped vibrator—without having to bring someone else into your bedroom.

2. *Magical wands*

These don't buzz, twirl, or pulsate, but they sure will get you pumped.

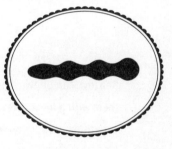

💜 **Glass wands.** Glass toys are exciting because they're pretty to look at and they're hard and very smooth at the same time. You can warm these toys up or cool them down, both of which allow you to explore different temperatures and sensations during your session, which can be very exciting.

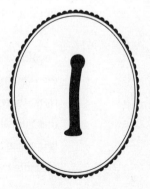

💜 **Silicone shafts.** Okay, fine, these are really called dildos. But *shaft* sounds so much sexier and more modern! These are typically graphic reproductions of male members, in a flexible silicone shape that you can ride on for internal joy, or rub against for external fun. They're awesome when used along with a C-Spot vibrator or your partner's touch. Your partner might also enjoy watching you enjoy a shaft—it's a huge visual turn-on.

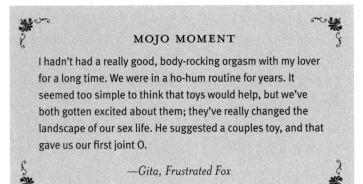

MOJO MOMENT

I hadn't had a really good, body-rocking orgasm with my lover for a long time. We were in a ho-hum routine for years. It seemed too simple to think that toys would help, but we've both gotten excited about them; they've really changed the landscape of our sex life. He suggested a couples toy, and that gave us our first joint O.

—*Gita, Frustrated Fox*

3. Couples toys

Sex toys can be twice as much fun when you share them with a lover. They inspire countless new variations in your sexy encounters, but they can also bring you closer as a couple. I always say that the couple that plays together stays together. Here are two core types of couples toys to consider:

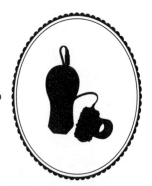

♥ **Couples rings.** If you're searching for the Big O during intercourse, then you need to add in a vibrating couples ring. This is how they work: there's a vibrating bullet that slides into a soft, stretchy ring that slides down his shaft, right to the base. Once that bullet is in place and you're on top, you're getting the additional C-Spot pleasure that'll help you reach orgasm during intercourse.

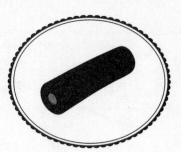

💜 **Pleasure sleeve.** This is a soft, pliable tube that typically has some kind of nubby texture on the interior; it slides down his entire shaft and adds sensation to your *handy* work. The sleeve grips, caresses, and stimulates his most sensitive part and makes you look like a pro. And not for nothing, using a sleeve can make things much easier for you.

WHAT'S THE BEST
FIRST TOY?

Honestly, the best starter toy is the one you see that instantly makes you feel comfortable and excited. Flip through catalogs or visit Bootyparlor.com. The photos of how it looks and the description of how it's meant to be used are all factors that will grab you, depending on your personality.

But in general, the best beginner toy is either a pocket rocket–style vibe or a modest-size classic vibrator. These are nice and simple and so easy to use. (The classic toy The Champ is everyone's favorite starter, and keeper, toy.) Whatever you choose, look for one where you can control the intensity, and consider seeking out a waterproof model so you have the option to use it in the shower. Enjoy!

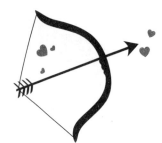

EXERCISE

Keep up
the 5-O Program

This week, add one item to your existing accessory collection. (And if you don't already have one, then this will be your first—congrats!) When you use it, get noisy! Vocalize what you're feeling as your pleasure becomes more and more intense and especially as that Big O pulses through your bod. It will bring a whole new sensory experience into the playground—and your pleasure will stick in your memory, giving you something to think about as you build up your anticipation next time.

MOJO MEMO:

Make a Love Kit

As a way to practice *layering* your turn-on accessories, I want you to create a sexy-experience kit of your own. Decide on a theme and go from there: it can be romantic, racy, pampering, all solo, or intended to be shared with a partner. Your Love Kit might include lingerie, a lip gloss, a special lubricant, chocolate body fondue, a whipper, a blindfold, a vibrator, a racy book . . . whatever it takes to create a six- to seven-piece kit that you can store in a pretty box in your closet. (If you already have items that work, great! If you prefer to add some new things, go shopping!) Every time you see the box, it will remind you that a sexy experience is seconds away.

I'm excited for you—you're going to be feeling good about your space and everything that you've learned about sexy accessories. (You're an expert on that subject now!) You've got other tasks coming up, but I hope that you'll be inspired to tinker with your other spaces—a car or office can be made into a mobile or off-site oasis with the right tweaks. In fact, that will be a perfect upkeep exercise for you to do on your own down the road: create new playgrounds!

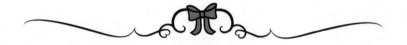

CONGRATULATIONS! AT THIS POINT IN YOUR MOJO MAKEOVER, YOUR EYES ARE OPEN TO THE SEXY IN EVERYDAY LIFE. GET READY TO LEARN HOW TO MASTER THE ART OF SEXY TALK AND SEE HOW IT CAN FURTHER INSPIRE SEXY EXPERIENCES BOTH INSIDE AND OUTSIDE THE BEDROOM. GET GOING— THE NEXT CHAPTER AWAITS!

CHAPTER THIRTEEN

The Art of Talking Dirty

THERE'S ANOTHER WAY TO EXPERIENCE A WELL-ROUNDED SENSE OF sexual satisfaction that we haven't touched on yet, but we're going to explore it intimately here: sexy talk. We worked on expressing desires in Chapter 10 as part of learning how to communicate what you want for more satisfying sex. But here, I'm talking about pure ear candy.

Sexy talk—also known as talking dirty—is a tool you can whip out to ratchet your heat up to a whole new level. By practicing it, you train yourself to be more assertive, which is empowering and a Mojo booster extraordinaire. I promise you'll love the way it adds sizzle to foreplay, which we'll also be getting down and dirty with in this chapter.

Sure, you may feel silly at first, and that's fine! Sex is often silly, funny, and dirty. Just remind yourself that it's a new thing to try as part of your mission to reach more frequent, more glorious orgasms!

If your initial reaction to talking dirty is fear, don't worry. I'm not trying to transform you into the phone sex operator of the month, but I do want you to be the sexiest, most authentic version of yourself, and this is part of that exploration. Using words that are comfortable to you will keep your confidence up—and there are plenty of ideas to try below, so you'll definitely find your place.

HOW TO TALK DIRTY TO YOURSELF

Practice makes perfect, and practicing on yourself can be ideal because you won't feel nervous as you might with a partner. (It also adds a new layer of seduction into your solo sessions!) An easy starting point is to simply say, "I like the way _____ feels" as you caress and care for yourself. It could be "innocent," like the way your bath sponge feels against your skin—or your nipples—in the tub, or how "sexy" it feels to massage lotion into your naked skin after.

Work on being more and more specific. Let your memory wander to the sexiest experiences you've ever had, or the ones you've always wanted to try. As you caress yourself, think of how a special lover once touched you or make up a story using a person you're secretly hot for. Or place yourself in a spot you find daring, like an elevator or bathroom stall, and build a mini-movie in your head, one where you feel the walls are close, clothes are being pulled off and unzipped, and the thrill of being discovered is all around. Incorporate your body, your hands, and toys, and let yourself go!

I'd like you to say these thoughts out loud, but if at first you feel best doing this in your mind, that's fine. Use a seductive voice (even in your head), enunciate the words, and sprinkle in some moans where it feels natural. You certainly know what you like and why, so say it! Once you have some racy dialogue in your head, you can play it back and bring even more excitement to your next sexy session.

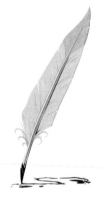

JOURNALING EXERCISE

"Talk" to Yourself

Lay some dirty talk on yourself during one of your sexy solo sessions, and then make notes about it in your journal by answering these questions:

❤ What approach did you take from the content above? Did you talk out loud?

❤ Did it feel funny at first? Or like second nature?

❤ Were you able to get into it?

❤ Did it bring newness and excitement to your sexy solo session?

HOW TO TALK DIRTY WITH A PARTNER

Honestly, saying what feels good or asking for what you want in a seductive manner is all it takes to be a smooth dirty talker. If you're not yet ready to hit your lover with something as graphic as *I love it when you go down on me*, then try *I love the way your tongue feels on my skin*. I'm telling you, *that* will set off a blast of arousal in your partner that will excite you both. If you're still not comfy, talk into a mirror. It's a good trick for giving a presentation and for sexy talk, too.

When you look at yourself and see and hear words coming out of your mouth, they become more natural. Body language—rubbing against your partner as you use your words—will contribute to the hot energy. So can whispering into a lover's ear. The heat of your breath and a few sultry words is incredibly scintillating. Turn on your partner with this simple phrase: *What do you want?* Dirty? Not on paper, but in a seductive moment, it will come off as naughty as a string of four-letter words, I promise!

MOJO MEMO:

A Word About Body Parts and Graphic Language

Using anatomical words or really graphic words to address body parts comes easily and comfortably to some women, but for many of us, saying, *Your cock is so hot!* just doesn't roll off the tongue. Say what feels right. Use "member" or "shaft" instead of "dick." And remember, the delivery is half of what makes your language lusty.

SEXY TALK 101

Here are a few basic approaches to get your sexy mouth moving. You'll see how easy and unintimidating this can be. Before you know it, you'll be *purring* sexy somethings like a pro.

💜 Approach 1: **Say what you're feeling.**

It's easy, I promise. You're just verbalizing the gorgeous sensations you're experiencing at that very moment. This is a great starting point if you're shy, and it's a little bit like cheering your lover on. In between your moans of pleasure, add in little touches like these:

> *You're so deep; it feels so good.*
> *I love putting my hands on your shaft; it's so thick and sexy.*
> *Mmm, it really turns me on when you touch me . . . right . . . there.*

💜 Approach 2: **Ask for more of what your lover is offering.**

It's a way to boost your partner's Mojo and encourage the moves *you'd* love more of so your bedmate can get you to that sweet O. Positive reinforcement will lead your lover to give you more of exactly what you're desiring.

> *Your fingers feel good on my G-Spot—keep moving just like that.*
> *You can go even harder . . . I like it that way.*
> *What you just did with your tongue was amazing.*
> *I'm getting close to my O . . . don't stop.*

TIP: Take the opportunity to physically drive home what you're verbalizing. For example, if you say, "You can go harder," grip onto your lover hard to pull him closer.

♥ **Approach 3: Describe what you're about to do.**

This can be a big turn-on and build anticipation in the moment. And of course, all this conversation should be going both ways between you two!

> *I'm going to lick your thighs so slowly.*
> *I'm going to tease the tip with little kisses and then take your shaft in my mouth.*
> *I'm going to touch myself with this toy . . . and I want you to watch.*
> *I'm going to give you the biggest, most explosive orgasm ever . . .*

♥ **Approach 4: Ask confident questions (that also compliment you in return)!**

The fact that you're self-assured about turning him on will be a turn-on for you both. These will definitely rope him into trying sexy talk along with you:

> *Do you like when my tongue is*
>   *on your shaft?*
> *You love that I love to be*
>   *spanked, yes?*
> *I wore my special outfit just for*
>   *you . . . Doesn't my ass look sexy?*

TIP: As you refer to one of your body parts, give him a tantalizing view of it—lick your tongue across your lips, shake your sexy bum—it invites him to touch you there.

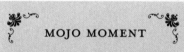

MOJO MOMENT

I had a hard time with the dirty-talk exercise, so I decided to read the fantasy I had written for another exercise out loud to my partner instead. It was a little hard at some points but felt good to read it. I think this could be a good way to start opening up in that way. If you're shy like me, I recommend it!

—Amy, Pleasure Virgin

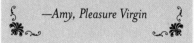

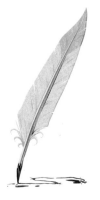

**JOURNALING
EXERCISE**

Talk to *Your* Partner!

During one of your partner sessions in the Big 5-O program, integrate talking dirty with your lover. Do some prep work based on the four approaches listed above, make notes, and get ready! Afterward, answer these questions:

❤ What approach did you take?

❤ Did it feel funny at first? Awkward? Were you nervous or raring to go?

❤ Once you got into it, how did it make you feel? Naughty? Turned on? More seductive? In control?

❤ Did it bring newness and excitement to your frisky encounter?

❤ How'd your partner react? Did he get into it and reciprocate?

SEXY TALK FROM AFAR

If you can't engage in live sexy talk right now, use it to your advantage and build anticipation for the next time you're face-to-face. That's what makes phone sex so awesome. The same for sexy texting, picture and video messaging, and naughty e-mails. They get you and your partner thinking about each other all day long and build anticipation for what's to come later. All that pent-up sexual energy makes for a supersonic love session—you'll want to rip each other's clothes off as soon as you're finally together. Ecstasy!

Common sense cautions

First, think of the surroundings where your
partner will receive any sort of sexy
communication. If it's on a large computer in
an open-plan office, a coworker might see an
incoming e-mail (for this reason be careful how
you word the subject line—I'd suggest some
hint that the info inside is for solo viewing).
The same applies to instant messages, photos,
and video clips. Of course, you need to trust
that the recipient is mature and respectful of you and won't plaster your business
all over the Internet or on his Facebook page. And for heaven's sake, double-
check the phone number or e-mail address before you hit SEND. (Never, ever
piggyback on an old e-mail—imagine you hit REPLY ALL by mistake?) And phones
do get lost . . . so remember anyone could view what you've sent.

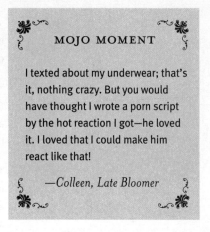

MOJO MOMENT

I texted about my underwear; that's
it, nothing crazy. But you would
have thought I wrote a porn script
by the hot reaction I got—he loved
it. I loved that I could make him
react like that!

—*Colleen, Late Bloomer*

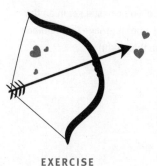

EXERCISE

Send a Sext Right Now!

❤ Be bold but brief.

A little mental stimulation goes a long way. In a text,
try, *Come home and rip my clothes off.* Or, *There's
chocolate by the bed; come home and feed me.*

❤ Put a sexy spin on a daily domesticity.

Video chat with your love interest and let him know
that when you sign off you'll be doing the dishes . . .

in a naughty outfit. Call and say that you'll pick up dinner . . . along with a can of whipped cream for later.

❤ Share what you're wearing.

E-mail that you'll be wearing special sexy panties today and you'll be thinking about your lover pulling them off that night.

❤ Tease, straight-up.

If your partner's on the way home, get into a towel and send a little video clip saying you're getting into a steamy shower . . . and you'll be waiting for him to kiss your fresh, clean skin when he gets home.

❤ Use timing to your advantage.

When your lover sends you a response to your sexy message, don't reply right away. It may be tempting to message right back, but drawing things out a bit will build anticipation.

❤ Sext yourself!

If you're not partnered up, you can still get in on the frisky fun. Send yourself a hot message that reminds you about a solo session that night!

MOJO MEMO:

Remember to Lean on Your Girlfriends!

Still feeling lost? Share ideas with your BFFs. When you meet for girls' night this week, you can help one another craft the few perfect lines. Doing this with your girls will normalize the experience and, in doing so, break through any hesitation you have about talking dirty with your partner. You might discover some things that you never knew your friends were into!

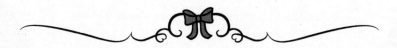

SO, WE'RE CRYSTAL CLEAR NOW THAT SEXY TALK (IN PERSON OR NOT) IS A DELICIOUS BUILDUP TO SEXUAL BLISS. BUT LET'S EXPAND ON THAT— IT'S TIME TO TRANSFORM YOUR FOREPLAY EXPERIENCES INTO SOMETHING MORE DARING, INTERESTING, AND SUPERBLY PLEASURABLE!

This Week's Mojo Mission

MASTERING YOUR MOJO!

The Mojo Makeover is gelling big-time now. You've worked so hard, learned so much, come so far! Your sexy self-confidence is boosted, and you're already seeing the results in your sex life. Your Mojo is now an integral part of your daily life—you're feeling it at work, at the gym, with friends, with your partner . . . both in and out of the bedroom.

GET READY TO

- ❤ Build anticipation and pleasure by making the most out of foreplay.

- ❤ Seduce your partner (or yourself) in smoking-hot lingerie.

- ❤ Create game-changing experiences by revealing and acting on your fantasies.

- ❤ Put everything into action with some sassy real-life flirting.

KEEP UP THE GOOD MOJO WORK!

Continue the Big 5-O this week and after the makeover is finished. You're going to find that, with everything you've learned and how you've evolved, your charged-up confidence and lit-up libido will lead you there naturally!

CHAPTER FOURTEEN

Focus on Foreplay

SEX ISN'T ABOUT ONLY THE END RESULT; IT'S ABOUT THE JOURNEY that builds up to the end result. Sometimes quickies can be passionate and erotic—being tossed onto a desk at your guy's office or locking yourself in a bathroom because you have to satisfy yourself *right now this second*. But foreplay can be an opportunity to connect, build intimacy, focus on the five senses, and build up anticipation for the Big O (or several orgasms in one sexy session!). I find that the newer the relationship, the more foreplay there is, but also that over time it shrinks and can become . . . well, dull. It can be your own rut or a partner's, in which case, opening the lines of communication and incorporating some raunchy (but directive) dirty talk will help spark variety and wake things back up. You should also tap into the foreplay pick-me-ups below. These will reinvigorate your together time and make you love foreplay in a whole new way. To start, I want you to think about the role foreplay plays in your life now.

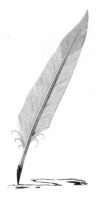

Your Current
State of Foreplay

To get your head wrapped around where you want to go—where you need to go—with foreplay in your love life, answer these questions in your journal. Be open and honest (as always), but don't let any negatives bring you down. That's not the point: writing down where your foreplay is will illuminate the possibilities for how easily you can change things up.

**JOURNALING
EXERCISE**

- Are you happy with it?

- Is it the same every time?

- How long does your foreplay usually last?

- What does it consist of?

- What do you want more of?

- What does he want more of?

FOREPLAY BOOSTERS:
EIGHT WAYS TO ENJOY THE SEX
BEFORE THE SEX

This is a starting point—each suggestion could spawn ten, twenty, or more additional ideas. Use these for inspiration, but in no way let this list limit your creativity!

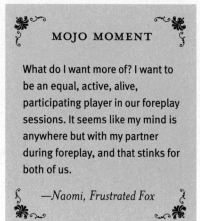

1. *Mental foreplay*

It is sometimes said that the human body's most erogenous zone is the mind. Practice some of the possibilities we've just covered, like e-messages or sexy talk. Visual stimulation like lingerie gets the mind racing, and so can erotic locations, like the elevator in your fantasy.

2. *Kisses of all kinds*

There are *so* many types of kisses, and so much you can *do* with kissing . . . on the lips, of course (deep passionate kisses rule!); on both your and his erogenous zones: neck, ears, wrists, nipples, breasts, inner thighs, back, behind the knees, the bum, even feet . . . and anything and everything between the legs. Think about creating a marathon makeout session by exploring some of these sexy smooches:

- ♥ **Butterfly kisses.** Light little flutters with your eyelashes that create a whisper-light touch on skin. Very sensual . . .

- ♥ **Eskimo kisses.** Using your nose to nudge your lover on the face, cheeks, all over the body, draping your hair across the skin as you go. It's a very primal nudge, very animal-like.

MOJO MOMENT

The ice-cube kisses were the most fun because of the intensity of the cold, and it added laughter to our session, which brought us to a whole new level of sexy.

—Rosalie, Adventure Seeker

- ❤ **Nibbling or light biting kisses.** Seductive nibbles can deliver exciting sensations. A little nip can really wake up the nerves and skin.

- ❤ **Upside-down kisses.** As we all remember from *Spider-Man,* these can be very sensual.

- ❤ **French kisses.** Either mad and passionate or slow and sexy, reconnecting with this kind of kissing can be really intimate.

- ❤ **Ice-cube kissing.** Putting an ice cube in your mouth and tracing it all over your lover's erogenous zones . . . hot!

3. Sensual touch

Massage is great for slowing down and reconnecting with your lover. It relieves stress and stimulates the senses instead of rushing into intercourse, and it's definitely worth the effort:

💜 **Use a good massage oil.** You want one with a smooth, nonsticky texture, something that has a good slip, but also absorbs into the skin so you don't feel sticky afterwards.

💜 **Warm it up.** Pour the oil into your palms and rub them together to increase the heat. Alternately, use a soy-based massage candle. Set the scene for seduction with the candle's glow, then blow out the flame and drizzle the warm oil onto bare skin for a uniquely intimate, exciting massage experience. (You get to fulfill the classic hot-wax fantasy without the fear of getting burned!)

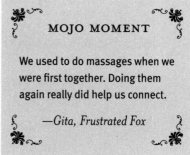

MOJO MOMENT

We used to do massages when we were first together. Doing them again really did help us connect.

—*Gita, Frustrated Fox*

💜 **Vary your moves.** Try gliding your hands, swirling, kneading. Your goal is to keep it sexy: this is not a sports massage.

💜 **Don't take turns in one session.** Massage doesn't always have to be a *your turn, my turn* kind of thing. I think the best system is *my day, your day* because then you're not thinking about having to "work" after you've received one.

💜 **Build steam.** At some point, the massage should transition into sexier places around your pleasure points. (Worth noting: Breasts and chests love being massaged! Having oil drizzled on them is a really sexy feeling.) To take *his* massage to the next erotic level, work into his inner thighs, lightly touch his johnson and jewels—but then go back to other parts, so that he craves your touch. It's not necessarily about going into full handy-work mode. You want to pace it out and just give a hint of what's next in your foreplay session.

4. Tickling

Most people hate aggressive tickling. It makes you want to punch your attacker, right? This is not the kind of tickling I'm suggesting. (Though some people do have a serious tickling fetish.)

- ❤ **Go easy-teasy.** What I'm suggesting here is the kind of tickling touch that feels like light feathers being dragged across the skin, simply prickling up those nerve endings on the surface, making your body want to reach up to the sensation and get more.

- ❤ **Use a ticklish toy.** I recommend any kind of feather tickler or wand here. Marabou is the softest and most angelic.

5. Scratching

Light scratching can feel seriously erotic on the skin.

- ❤ **Keep it light!** I'm not suggesting scratching to draw blood here, of course. So first and foremost, check each other's nails to make

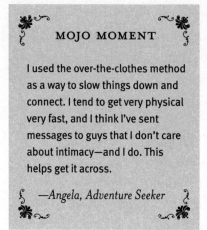

sure there are no jagged edges. Experiment from a light tickling scratch to a hungrier scratch down the back. The sensation is soothing and provocative all at once.

6. *Manual pleasure*

Manual stimulation is truly fantastic foreplay because it can deliver sweet satisfaction in ways that penetration simply can't.

- ♥ **Start with your clothes on.** No one likes it when her lover goes straight for the bull's-eye. So encourage a slow warm-up—gently glide your lover's hand on the outside of your jeans first, and then let your partner continue over your panties. Eventually, slide his hands underneath them. At that point, you'll be getting warm and will be lusting for his touch on your bare skin.

- ♥ **Work up to the G-Spot.** As you get hot and bothered, he can seek out your G-Spot with one hand and work your C-Spot simultaneously with the other. Or if he's adept, he can tend to both spots at once using one hand—that can really drive you to an incredible place.

💜 **Let him see your body.** As you start to stimulate his body, let him see yours. A clear view of your naked breasts as you handle his shaft will really amp up his excitement. (Men are very visual creatures!) Use a pleasure sleeve if you like, but don't take him all the way just yet. Lower your breasts against him; the softness of your sexy bust coupled with the intensity of your grip will arouse him intensely.

💜 **Explore his A-Spot.** This can be a huge turn-on for a man and really heighten his orgasm. You want to take that slowly and make sure he's comfortable with it—either by asking him or by touching a little bit and reading his body language in response. Remember to always use lubricant with A-Spot play!

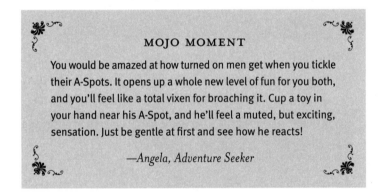

MOJO MOMENT

You would be amazed at how turned on men get when you tickle their A-Spots. It opens up a whole new level of fun for you both, and you'll feel like a total vixen for broaching it. Cup a toy in your hand near his A-Spot, and he'll feel a muted, but exciting, sensation. Just be gentle at first and see how he reacts!

—*Angela, Adventure Seeker*

7. Oral stimulation

If you embrace oral stimulation by both giving and receiving, it builds intimacy, it's hugely stimulating, and can lead to *incredible* orgasms. Receiving oral sex is one of the best ways to really release your sexiest self. You're allowing your lover very intimate access to the center of your sex and that's powerful; it's very goddess-like, so really embrace that sense and let yourself be worshipped.

💜 **Relax.** When you're receiving, you need to let go of any self-conscious feelings you have. If you're concerned about tastes or smells, showering ahead (or keeping feminine wipes handy) works for both sexes. So does yummy-flavored lubricant or female-friendly body toppings.

💜 **Convey your delight.** You'll want to give plenty of signals to your lover on what feels good. (Pushing forward or rocking with your partner's motions is always a good signal that you're enjoying something.) Be sure to verbalize it with some sexy talk, too.

💜 **Double your pleasure.** Adding in manual stimulation can be incredibly pleasurable, so much so that it might finish you off then and there. For the sake of prolonged foreplay, be strong and back it off if it boosts your pleasure toward the O zone too quickly.

💜 **Feel confident when giving.** A guy will find great pleasure receiving oral pretty much any which way you deliver it, and that alone should make anyone feel like the Queen of Sheba. Confidence and enthusiasm (why not be enthusiastic?) are key!

💜 **Put on a show for him.** Use lots of eye contact and exaggerate every motion. Let him feel and see the slow sliding of your lips and tongue up and down his shaft. You'll have fun and feel so empowered knowing that you're really turning him on.

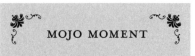

MOJO MOMENT

My husband is very large, and I'd gag on him thinking I needed to take on his whole shaft! This got so bad that I'd simply stopped giving him oral sex. It caused a divide—he missed it, and I felt frustrated that I couldn't pleasure him that way. Now that I'm using my hands, as well, I feel so much more in control and so much more confident in my ability to pleasure him. I also practice my yoga breathing during oral—in and out through my nose—it relaxes me even further and makes a huge difference, too!

—*Gita, Frustrated Fox*

♥ **Avoid gagging.** Add your hands to the base of his shaft to control the amount you prefer to take in your mouth. This gives you the control you desire to enjoy the experience, and the added touch also feels super good for him.

♥ **Touch the jewels.** The shaft is the main player, but the boys need love, too—the bonus sensation will really turn him on. Gentle tickling, kissing, and even blowing are good options to start here.

♥ **Get sloppy.** Wear red lipstick and let it smear a little on your face during your session. Messy is sexy.

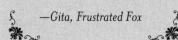 **Use your mouth to its full ability.** Humming, sucking, being attentive to the underside of the tip, twisting your mouth (or hand), and moving your tongue and tongue tip around will be much appreciated.

8. *Unlimited options!*

Once you put your focus on foreplay, you'll see the unlimited options that exist for you. Here are just a few others to consider:

- ♥ **Show off your passion.** For some, PDA is highly erotic foreplay. I don't mean aggressively squeezing his package on a city street. I mean engaging in more sweet affection more often: holding hands, kissing over dinner, touching each other's faces . . . Little acts like these make each of you feel wanted.

- ♥ **Get your adrenaline pumping.** Personal fantasies about particular locations or activities that you find highly stimulating can be quite a turn-on. This could be skydiving, rock climbing, or hitting a theme park as a couple. Get your blood pumping and let the thrill of your adventure be mental foreplay for what's to come later.

- ♥ **Play a role.** Playing out a fantasy, perhaps with the help of ornate costumes and props, can be a thrilling act of foreplay for some. You know who you are—more power to you!

THE FOREPLAY CHALLENGE!

It's time to take what you know—and what you want—from foreplay and put it into action with the Foreplay Challenge.

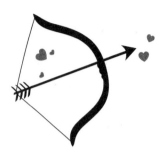

EXERCISE

The Foreplay Challenge *for* Couples

Are you partnered up? Grab your lover and try two of these experiences, or any of the others you've learned earlier in this chapter:

1. HAVE A MARATHON. Incorporate oral fun, toys, touches, pinches, positions, and sexy videos. See how many things you can include before orgasm.

2. TRY THE NO-PENETRATION CHALLENGE. Your challenge is to commit to reaching an orgasm without intercourse. It encourages you to explore types of foreplay where your partner brings you to an O first, and then you bring your partner there. Or you can explore penetration-free ways to reach the O at the same time.

3. INDULGE IN A SENSUAL NINE-AND-A-HALF-WEEKS EXPERIENCE. This is food for foreplay. Feed cut-up fruit dipped in chocolate to each other to excite the senses. Better yet, take turns blindfolding each other and guessing what it is you're being fed. Also, try using a blindfold and drizzling things on each other's bodies, like Booty Parlor's kissable body topping Skin Honey. With a blindfold on, the anticipation of where it's being drizzled next (and the feeling of when it first strikes the skin) will be very exhilarating.

4. DO A DAYLONG FOREPLAY. Starting in the morning with sexy love notes and sending a text to build anticipation, meet for dinner wearing vibrating panties, and then finally . . . when you get home . . . go for the goal! Go crazy on each other!

MOJO MOMENT

Once I got over my OCD about cleanliness and having food on my body, I really got into this. We experimented getting messy and sexy with fruits, chocolate, peanut butter, ice cream, and even champagne! We used ice cubes, as well—the way they numb the skin was totally kinky. I loved it so much I ended up using ice for a solo session the next day!

—*Rosalie, Adventure Seeker*

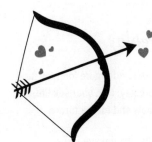

The *Foreplay* Challenge *for Singles*

Are you a solo player? Try two of these self-satisfying moves or pick one from the list of boosters earlier in the chapter.

EXERCISE

1. **MAKE IT ABOUT ENDURANCE.** Bring yourself up and down using a toy with multiple settings. Focus on not having an orgasm, drawing it out till you absolutely must climax.

2. **TOUCH YOURSELF IN A FOREIGN WAY.** A lot of women go straight for the motion they love. This challenge is about enjoying your body first. Clasp your breasts, run your hands through your hair, explore your body, then move towards the strokes and sensations that you love because they get you there.

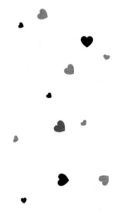

3. DANCE AND STRIP FOR YOURSELF. It can be a huge turn-on to watch yourself in the mirror. It can be a racy and intimate experience, especially because it's private—it's for your eyes only!

4. WARM UP YOUR MIND. When you're in a morning meeting, allow yourself to think about the big orgasm you're going to give yourself later that day. Build anticipation in your mind so when you get home, you're ready to ravish yourself.

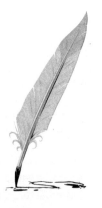

Your New Improved State of Foreplay

Now that you've worked on how to add more foreplay (and more enjoyable varieties of foreplay) into your sex life, it's time to note its impact, both now and for the future.

JOURNALING EXERCISE

- Which foreplay boosters and tips did you try?

- Where they a hit? Why?

- How long did your foreplay last? Are you pleased with that?

- Any flops? Why?

- What other tips are you tempted to try? Why?

- What do you want more of now?

- What does he want more of now?

MOJO MOMENT

I feel I look super awkward when I dance in the mirror, and it makes me laugh. But I'm feeling sexier inside, and more confident and seductive. I know I have the potential to rock this dancing and stripping for myself thing with some practice. I've already developed a signature move that is sort of like a rodeo arm, and I yell, woooh! I combine this move with a sexy hip roll. It's amazing. It made me laugh; it turned me on. I highly recommend it.

—*Gia, Pleasure Virgin*

Whew! I know this has been a *lot* of juicy info, and no question, you've picked up new Mojo tools that further help you express your sexy self—and that will bring you even more sexual confidence, excitement, and intimacy. Enjoy putting everything into action!

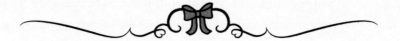

NOW THAT YOU'VE DISCOVERED NEW WAYS TO BUILD ANTICIPATION IN YOUR SEXY LIFESTYLE, IT'S TIME TO STEP INTO SOMETHING MORE . . . INTIMATE. IN THE NEXT CHAPTER I'M GOING TO TELL YOU HOW TO FEEL (AND MOVE) LIKE A SEDUCTIVE GODDESS IN LINGERIE SO YOU *OWN* THE MOMENT THAT YOU'RE WEARING IT— AND THE MOMENT AFTER IT'S OFF!

CHAPTER FIFTEEN

Lingerie for Seduction

I N WEEK TWO OF THE MOJO MAKEOVER, WE COVERED FUNCTIONAL, pretty daytime skivvies, and how wearing things that fit well, in fabrics and designs you love, can be a treat that boosts your confidence every day. But that's not all you need to know about underpinnings. It's time to go to the next level and learn how to use sexy underthings to enhance your love life—we're going to explore the joys of seduction-specific pieces, including how to move in them to create risqué moments for enjoyment with or without a partner.

To be clear, in this chapter, when I refer to lingerie, I'm talking about the racier stuff that you may already own and that you pull out for special nights. That said, if you *do* save your racy gear for special times, I want to break you out of that habit right now. Why not wear something naughty during the day? Hiding something daring under work outfits or jeans can be one of the sexiest secret weapons in your Mojo bag of tricks. You'll be stashing a sexy secret, feeling an inner effervescence that bubbles up as little smiles during the day, leaving others to wonder, *Ooh, what's she got going on*?

OUTFITTING YOURSELF
TO LOOK AND FEEL YOUR BEST

For practical reasons, most of the time, we save our sexiest lingerie for the bedroom. (Stripper shoes generally won't cut it at work.) When I outfit myself specifically for seduction encounters, I like to think of it as playing dress-up. You have *so* many sexy sides you can uncover and express through lingerie. You may be feeling really romantic and soft and innocent, you may be feeling strong and powerful and naughty, or you may be feeling as though you completely want to lose yourself in a fantasy look.

Dressing up in full seduction gear can give you a sense of freedom and mystery. It can inspire you to abandon your inhibitions and cut loose, opening yourself up to creative new things. It can allow you to transform routine sex into a creative playground. While a full lingerie getup may not become your routine gear every time you get busy, make an effort to integrate it once a week or once every two weeks. It will come to be an extra special indulgence. Remember, lingerie isn't "for him." Of course, your lover will benefit from the visual feast you provide him. But it's really for *you*! When you get an eyeful of your seductive power in lingerie, you'll get turned on and realize, *Wow, am I sexy!*

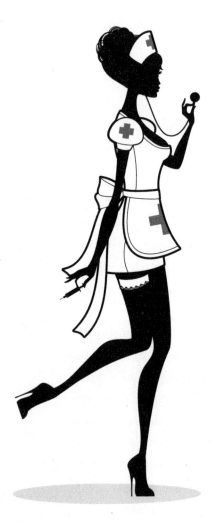

IS THERE A NAUGHTY NURSE IN THE HOUSE?

It's fun to dress up in a costume, and compared to some pieces of lingerie, it can be a steal! For under thirty dollars you can get a complete dishy ensemble like a French maid or naughty nurse, and trust me, it's fun. If you've never done it before, it might feel weird the first few times, but it's very freeing, especially within a long-term relationship that needs some spice. (Sexy costumes also cover more of you up than many pieces of lingerie. For example, most maid costumes have an apron and cap sleeves, and some of us feel more confident that way.) You can find yourself really getting into a role, like a sexy schoolteacher. Ask your lover to play the pupil and bring in a notebook and grade his homework assignments! It's a way to let loose. And it's really kinky, which can feel adventurous and empowering. There are plenty of costumes that allow guys to role-play, too. I'm a fan of rogue pirates, bad cops, and soccer players myself!

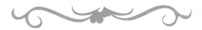

LET'S GET YOUR
SEDUCTIVE COLLECTION STARTED!

When it comes to risqué lingerie, I love wearing a full set where the items are all part of one look and convey a specific vibe, like daring vixen or a romantic nymph. I always get ready in a room separate from my hubbie so that I can make an entrance. I highly recommend you do the same because it really adds to the moment. Plus, it gives you the time to connect with yourself in the mirror, and even do your seductive beauty rituals to pump up your sexy self-confidence.

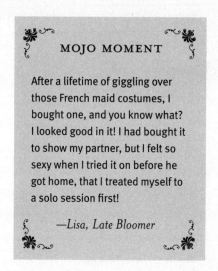

MOJO MOMENT

After a lifetime of giggling over those French maid costumes, I bought one, and you know what? I looked good in it! I had bought it to show my partner, but I felt so sexy when I tried it on before he got home, that I treated myself to a solo session first!

—*Lisa, Late Bloomer*

A simple look to start with is a bra, panties, garter belt, and stockings. You can buy an ensemble that's a perfect matched set or pull one together piece by piece with coordinated colors and fabrics, according to what flatters your assets the most. Some food for thought:

Bras

Get creative with see-through fabrics, cups that are cut low to reveal a peek of your nipples, cups that unsnap to reveal your breasts, cupless bras that expose the girls and just give some underwire push-up. Look for frills, ruffles, bows, scallops, deep cleavage, even marabou poufs on the nipple—really, any kind of highly sexy bra that you wouldn't (or actually couldn't) wear to work. Or skip the bra and try glittery nipple pasties or nipple tassels instead!

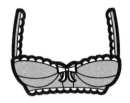

Panties

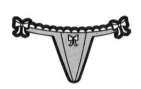

Think alluring details, like cutouts, peekaboo elements, and crotchless styles (which I recommend keeping on while you receive oral pleasure—this is seriously sexy for your lover and even sexier for you. Feeling his kisses and the fabric on your skin is electrifying.). Consider panties that are completely sheer, ones with ruffles that dance off the hips, or ones with revealing backside cleavage. Find a pair that is held up by pretty ribbons that tie at your hips . . . and can be untied to reveal your naked bod. There are tons and tons of sexy, sexy styles. The key is that they coordinate with other pieces of your lingerie outfit so you have the effect of a set.

Garters

If you've never worn a garter and stockings, you're in for a treat. These are such exciting additions to your lingerie outfit. They add a dash of sexiness, fantasy, and definite naughtiness. Garter belts cinch around your waist or hips, and have four small dangling straps that

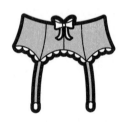

you latch on to stockings. The belt emphasizes your curves and the seductive straps draw attention to your gams. Stockings are a great way to flaunt and flirt with your legs. If a garter belt really isn't your thing, there are plenty of sexy panties that have built-in stocking straps, so you can still work your thigh-highs!

TIP: Put your garters and stockings on first, and then pull up your panties. This way, your lover can pull off your undies and your garters will still be in place . . . leaving you a vision of total sex appeal. It's very frisky, very daring, and altogether a total thrill!

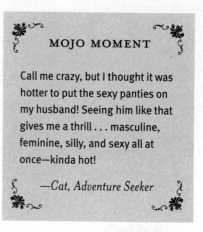

MOJO MOMENT

Call me crazy, but I thought it was hotter to put the sexy panties on my husband! Seeing him like that gives me a thrill . . . masculine, feminine, silly, and sexy all at once—kinda hot!

—*Cat, Adventure Seeker*

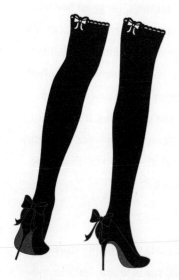

Thigh-high stockings

You'll need these to go with your garters, of course. There are *so* many styles to play with! Fishnets, which have a diamond pattern (if you have generous thighs, a closer-knit fishnet will be more flattering than wide-open ones; although the wide ones have a certain racy factor that's hot); sheers with or without back seams; striped; floral; wet-looking latex stockings . . . the list goes on. My personal favorite is a pair of sheer thigh-highs in a pale skin tone with a black snake winding its way up the back of each leg. They're just *out there*, naughty, and super powerful all at once. You can find stockings that require the garter straps to hold them up, but some thigh-highs have elastic bands at the top that hug your legs and hold them up—no garter required. They can still be clipped into your garter, but they look awesome alone. The softer your thighs, the more a thigh-high's elastic will press into them (like the dreaded muffin top, but on your legs), so that's something to consider when you're deciding which to buy. I tend not to skimp when I'm shopping for these, specifically for that reason. The more luxurious and high quality your stockings are, the less muffin-top leg you'll have! The main purpose here is to encourage you to feel great, so say no to anything that makes you feel self-conscious.

Heels

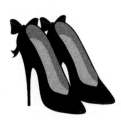

Once your feet are clad in stockings, I suggest finishing the look with a sexy heel. The classic heeled slipper with a fluffy marabou pouf is fun and very provocative. That's just one idea. Your fantasy footwear might be a sky-high stiletto pump or a Lucite stripper shoe or a thigh-high platform boot! And while it's hot for a lover to remove your shoes, it's quite erotic if you leave them on for the entire session. Not only does it add a naughty feel to the experience, the heels make your legs look awesome the whole time, which will then make you feel awesome about your bod.

The lingerie list goes on!

If you prefer a different kind of look, all it takes is a visit to a lingerie store or Internet site to see all sorts of possibilities that will speak to you. Teddies and baby dolls can be tight, flowing, see-through, or lace-up. Some offer built-in bust support and some don't. Corsets and waist cinchers celebrate a female hourglass shape (and can encourage one no matter what your size or shape is!).

Pieces that skim past the hips offer coverage and a peekaboo flirtiness at once. I have a skirted garter belt (literally a micromini with garters) that I love, especially if I'm feeling a touch of PMS bloat. It smooths my stomach and looks hot at the same time—what's not to love?

BORROWED FROM BURLESQUE:
THREE MOVES THAT
ANYONE CAN MASTER

How you hold yourself when wearing seductive lingerie is just as important as wearing the lingerie itself. In fact, one of the reasons that many women fear this type of lingerie is because they're unsure of how to work it! But not too worry: these three maneuvers will have you working it with a level of confidence you didn't even know you had.

1. *The Slow Walk*

Every woman's high-heeled walk will be different. Some women slink, some prance, and some have a showgirl stomp that's all about business. I encourage you to practice in front of a mirror until you discover what's right for you. Once you have it, you'll feel an amazing sense of

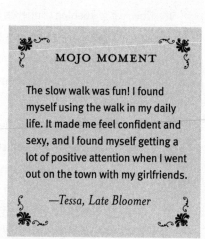

MOJO MOMENT

The slow walk was fun! I found myself using the walk in my daily life. It made me feel confident and sexy, and I found myself getting a lot of positive attention when I went out on the town with my girlfriends.

—Tessa, Late Bloomer

confidence that you'll carry with you, both inside and out of the bedroom. A couple basic tips:

💜 Engage your core for stability. Engaging your abdominals and back muscles will help you feel more solid on your heels.

💜 Draw your shoulders back, so that your bust juts forward. This will definitely throw off your center of gravity at the beginning, so just stand there and shift back and forth until you find that center again. It looks hot, so definitely practice until you nail it down.

💜 Your seductive, shoulder-back posture will naturally cause your bum to curve out behind you. Don't fight it—it helps you maintain balance!

💜 Now, while keeping your eyes forward on your lover, put one foot right in front of the other, in a heel-ball-toe, heel-ball-toe rhythm. Do it as if you were walking on a straight thin line. Your hips and shoulders will naturally gyrate as you cross one leg in front of the other, and that's very, very seductive. (When you're comfortable with the basic walk, experiment with a bit more bounce, a tiny little kickback with each step, let your arms sway behind your body, or place your hands on your hips.)

💜 Once you reach your partner, slowly lean down so your breasts are grazing his face and softly caress his hair or jaw or shoulders.

Then let the kissing and nibbling begin—or, add the Twist and
Dip below.

2. *The Twist and Dip*

For this you need to start by standing close to and facing your partner. Your lover
should be sitting on a bed, chair, or couch.

- ♥ **Run your hands through his hair and nuzzle his face into your
  bosom.** Then give his head a little toss back and prepare for your
  move: pull your shoulders back and set your feet slightly apart.

- ♥ **With your hands on his shoulders, slightly twist your waist so
  that your hips and knees swivel to one side.** (Your head and
  shoulders should still be facing him.)

- ♥ **Then, get low.** Start to bend your knees, engaging your thigh
  muscles with control and dip, dip, dip down until you can't dip
  any farther. This will place you in between his legs, where he'll be
  getting very aroused. Keep your shoulders back and your hands
  somewhere on his body to stabilize yourself.

- ♥ **Next, it's up to you whether you want to stay there, but I
  recommend getting back up:** slowly, slowly rise up, with your
  hands on his thighs, giving him a closeup eyeful of each body
  part as you move up. Repeat the dip, and tease him some more!

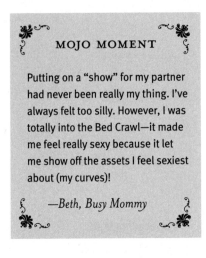

3. The Bed Crawl

This one is really fun; it puts you on center stage to show yourself off, and it's *super* simple. Crawl across the surface of the bed using your forearms to prop you up slightly. (You're not dragging yourself; it's more like a slow, slithering glide.) Skim your boobs just above the surface as you move onto the bed . . . Gyrate as though you were a sexy serpent goddess. Pop up your curvy bum, toss your hair, and use your shoulder and waist undulations with every move. It can be a very carnal thrill. Playing some sexy music can make it feel even more seductive. Anyone remember Duran Duran's "Hungry Like the Wolf" video? Look it up on the Internet—you'll be inspired!

UNDRESSING TIP:
HOW TO TAKE IT OFF LIKE A PRO

It can at times feel awkward to peel off your panties in front of someone else. (How many movies have you seen that made a mockery of the fumbling that can happen with the removal of a bra?) There is an art to taking it all off, but it boils down to three words: *Be. A. Tease.* Draw the moment out to build anticipation.

♥ Instead of just unclasping your bra, slide one finger under the shoulder straps and slowly push each off, one at a time.

Expose a bit more of your breast, but not the complete set yet. It's sexier to look half-dressed for a little bit. Hold the bra with one hand and slide the other hand's fingers to the clasp, release it, and then gingerly remove your bra. Make a show of dropping it to the floor.

♥ **Pull your panties down just a hint, teasing, playing with the edges, but then pull them back up.** Now, lie back, arch your lower back to accentuate your waist, and suggest *he* peel them off you. Slightly lift your hips so they don't get caught on your bum, then lay back and lift your forelegs up. Keep them together with pointed toes. Allow him to pull your panties completely off. Or flick them off from your toes and let them go flying across the room!

♥ **For intricate back-closure items, like a corset with hooks or laces, turn to give your lover a view of your fingers slowly, methodically undoing the cinches.** Or use your best enticing voice and ask him to help. Then slowly gyrate your upper body as he works (like a belly dancer's movements but in a more erotic, super slow motion).

♥ **Slip tops (or flowing teddies and baby dolls) should *slip* down your body.** Remove these while standing up, and make eye contact the entire time with your partner. Use a finger to glide off each shoulder strap, one at a time. Hold the slip up loosely with one arm and retrace the straps' path with light finger strokes to

keep his eyes riveted. Then—just like that—release your arm so
the gown drops down and puddles around your feet.

♥ **Removing stockings?** Keep your heels on and stand up with one
leg propped on a chair or the bed frame (not the mattress—it'll
make you too wobbly). Slowly undo the garter clips, and then roll
the stocking down your leg, pausing every few moments to caress
your thigh, until the stocking is by your calf. Twist around to sit on
the bed, and allow him to finish the job and remove your shoe and
stocking from your pointed foot. Then repeat with the other leg. I
have seen some incredible burlesque dancers remove their stockings
in the most unbelievable ways. Search YouTube for inspiration!

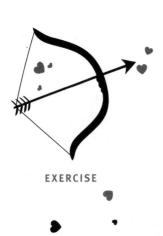

EXERCISE

Get Moving in the Mirror!

It's time to get your body and confidence prepped to
step into the lingerie you've just learned about. If you've
never experienced the joy of mirror dancing, it's about
time you did. What is it? It's a ritual—of course!—that
puts you in touch with the way your body naturally
moves and tunes you in to how it feels to move. Plus, it
helps you to adore your body in a whole new way. All you
need to do is turn on some music, dim the lights for a
seductive mood, plant yourself in front of a full-length
mirror, and move.

When I do my own mirror dancing sessions, I love to
dress up. Depending on my mood, I'll wear a low-cut wrap

dress and a sexy pair of heels; other times I'm barefoot in a cute pair of ruffled boy-short panties and a matching bralette. And if I'm feeling bloated and miserable, I'll still do it, but just in leggings and a tank. I want you to do it in your seductive lingerie the first few times. It will help you connect with the come-hither look and moves. After that, what you wear is up to you, but I encourage you to experiment with outfits so you can see different results each time.

A NOTE ABOUT MUSIC: Choose what feels right, but aim for a mix, to keep things varied (and fun). Try fun poppy tunes, see how some sexy songs work for you, and maybe even give some old-school favorites a spin. Trust me when I say you're going to enjoy this so much you'll want to set a weekly date with yourself. And you should!

Get Your Groove on—Starter Tips

💜 Create a sexy aura—dim the lights and have great music on hand, and don't forget props, like a feather boa or satin gloves.

💜 Use slow movements to get in tune with how strong you really are—it takes more strength to move slowly. Resist the impulse to immediately dance fast and wild.

💜 Feel the music and let your body flow along with the beat, be it just swaying your shoulders at first, stepping side to side, or gliding your arms through the air.

💜 Try smiling at yourself and even hamming it up with a pursed pucker, or licking your lips, or sucking a finger like a music video vixen—it'll help loosen you up.

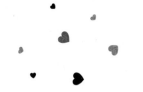

❤ Introduce some more-sensual movements, like winding your hips in a slow circle or slow-motion pelvic thrusts or both.

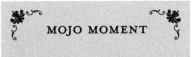

MOJO MOMENT

I wasn't sure if I would like mirror dancing, but the music is key. I just let it set the rhythm, and I got lost in it. All that practice gave me the confidence to show off my moves to my partner. He went wild for it, and that made me feel powerful.

—*Amy, Pleasure Virgin*

❤ Start running your hands over your body. Push your juicy butt out, shake it slowly from side to side, give it a little smack with the palm of your hand, all the while keeping your eyes closed or gazing at yourself in the mirror.

❤ Touch your breasts, your stomach, and run your hands through your hair. Imagine someone else's hands are on you (or even two other people's hands) joining in.

❤ Don't focus too hard on acting sexy, because you'll be distracted. Above all, enjoy yourself!

TEN SEXY TUNES FOR MIRROR DANCING

From my iPod to your ears—this is a fun varied mix, and some songs are a bit wild, but I can always find a song on my trusty list that matches my mood and gets me revved up!

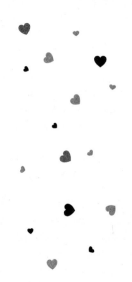

1. "Dance in the Dark" by Lady Gaga
2. "Closer" by Nine Inch Nails (it's a naughty one!)
3. "Love to Love You Baby" by Donna Summer
4. "Justify My Love" by Madonna
5. "American Boy" by Estelle featuring Kanye West
6. "Sexy MF" by Prince
7. "Candy Shop" by 50 Cent
8. "I'm a Slave 4 U" by Britney Spears
9. "Hey Sexy Lady" by Shaggy
10. "Love in an Elevator" by Aerosmith

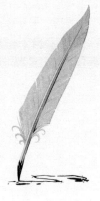

**JOURNALING
EXERCISE**

Did Mirror Dancing Move You?

In your journal, I want you to express your feelings about mirror dancing in your seductive lingerie. This exercise was a culmination of so many things that you've learned in this journey—reflect on that and give yourself tons of credit. It was a real "moment" for you . . . where you let go of inhibitions about your body, soaked up your sexy bedroom environment, wooed yourself, and let your inner and outer confidence shine through!

It's fun to dress up and to see yourself in a new light or to share that vision with a lover. Keep up the sexy dancing and update your iPod regularly with songs that inspire you to get it going with your body! It's one of many ways you can pay extra attention to yourself, and anytime you do that, your sexual inner self—your Mojo—gives back again and again.

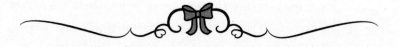

WE'RE MOVING FROM EXPLORING LINGERIE AND
MOVEMENT TO EXPLORING FANTASIES. OH, YES!
IN THE NEXT CHAPTER, WE'LL BE GOING TO PLACES
YOU NEVER THOUGHT YOU'D DARE . . . BUT TRUST ME—
YOU'RE MORE THAN READY!

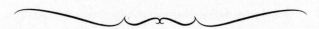

CHAPTER SIXTEEN

Exploring Fantasies

NOW THAT YOU'VE HIT A SEXY STRIDE IN YOUR MAKEOVER, IT'S time to explore your fantasies! Every one of us has them—what differs is the extent to which we allow ourselves to nurture them. I have found that many women allow themselves to have only fleeting fantasies, perhaps because they still haven't given themselves the permission to be fully realized sexual beings—they're afraid they'll be judged or that it's not ladylike. Well, I'm giving you permission to give *yourself* permission to fully engage your innermost fantasies. It's a key part of releasing that inner vixen and embracing your Mojo.

Having fantasies and learning how to share them can nourish your relationships, build intimacy, and increase the excitement tenfold. If you're single, having a rich fantasy life can make your solo sessions extra steamy and fresh. By allowing your thoughts to go absolutely anywhere, you'll be adding more layers to your sexual personality. Giving yourself permission to let those different "personalities" come out to play leads to feeling more confident in your sexiness, in your desires, and in knowing what you want—and isn't that a fabulous place to be?

A main exercise in this chapter is to write a fantasy. I want you to develop the imaginary story line and put yourself in a key role. Then I would like you to share your fantasy with a partner. I'll help you find your way—we'll practice how to think in fantasy mode and we'll explore the best ways to bring the subject up to a partner so you're confident about what you reveal. And you know what? Keeping it to yourself is an option, too.

Get excited. You're going to find out how fantasies can enrich your sex life.

IDENTIFY AND EMBRACE
YOUR HIDDEN DESIRES

There's no such thing as fantasies that are too tame or too "out there." They don't have to have anything to do with reality! Just because you fantasize about ravaging your boyfriend's best friend doesn't mean you're betraying your guy or that you love him less. Similarly, if you date men, yet the thought of a threesome including another woman turns you on, that doesn't mean you're unsure of your sexual orientation. It's really about fun and mental freedom. There's a whole world of erotic thoughts out there just waiting to be discovered by you.

Rate these fantasies!

A good starting point in this exploration is to let your mind travel through scores of steamy scenarios. Below, I've collected a bunch for your reading pleasure.

They're some of the most common fantasies I hear about from women. Eyeball them and circle one of the hearts to rate each one as either *cool, warm, hot, sizzling,* or *out of this world*. Doing so will reveal the types that turn you on and will steer your thoughts in the right mind-blowing direction.

1. ROLE-PLAYING

Acting out the role of a sexy character lets you and your lover step away from your traditional day-to-day lives and discover spicy new sexual possibilities. It allows the wild thing that's always been inside to take center stage. Whether you choose to be a night nurse on call with her doctor (he has to perform a full examination of your body); a schoolgirl with her professor (he'll give you good grades on your "skills" or send you to detention with a spanking); a French maid with her housemaster (*Oops*, you dropped the feather duster right by his feet!); a gangster with her mob boss (*My, what a big gun you have!*); or a call girl and her client (à la *Pretty Woman*, or something darker); role-playing fantasies are fun and ripe with storylines for you to enact time and time again.

2. SEX IN PUBLIC SPACES (OR ANY PLACE YOU MIGHT GET CAUGHT)

You secretly crave exhibitionism. The thought of being interrupted by a stranger, or watched by someone while you're in the act, or doing something naughty in a place you shouldn't be stirs something hot inside of you. Imagine wearing crotchless panties to a club and finding a dark corner where he presses you up against the wall and slips inside while throngs of people undulate just a few feet away on the dance

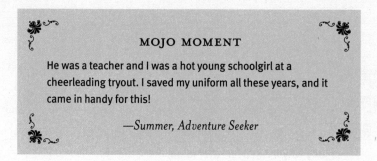

floor. Or you might get a thrill from the possibility of getting caught in
the act . . . like joining the mile-high club in a high-turbulence scenario,
sneaking into the back of an SUV in the middle of the day, or doing it
in the office storage room, skirt hiked, racing to finish your frisky
business before someone comes in.

3. BONDING . . . BEING TIED UP OR TYING SOMEONE ELSE UP

There's something exhilarating about being submissive (when you're
with someone you trust, that is). You're tied up, unable to move, but *so*
able to writhe your aroused body around, and you have no choice but
to succumb to your lover's kisses—anywhere he wants to plant them.
Every sense feels heightened; every touch, a bigger thrill. Wrists and
ankles, tied with silk scarves or bonding tape or neck ties—all of these
can be put to use. Alternatively, you might get a thrill out of tying him
up and having *your* way.

4. ONE-NIGHT STAND WITH A STRANGER

The no-strings-attached, I-don't-want-your-number-and-I'm-definitely-
not-going-to-give you-mine kind of passionate night. You meet him in a

dark sexy bar or on a subway car and then head to your apartment. You have a drink. You put on music. And you go at it—a night of wild, uninhibited, totally uncommitted, hungry sex with a stunning stranger. In imaginary fantasy land, there's no worrying about STDs or creeps . . . that's why it can be so awesome!

5. THREESOMES . . . OR MORE

Can you see yourself being seduced by two hot guys? Another couple? Maybe even two bodacious women? Or maybe you'd like to watch others get it on. There are so many combinations—of people and positions—to dream about when you're fantasizing about more than one bedmate. Anyway you fashion it, it's naughty and thrilling. All those arms, legs, lips, and extra attention being directed toward your pleasure. One of the more common fantasies I hear about is the experience of being serviced by two men at once—double penetration is *oh so* taboo, but *oh* such a turn-on to many women!

6. FETISHES

Nothing should be off limits in your fantasies. Some people adore feet or have stocking fetishes or lust after leather bondage gear, latex body stockings, spanking, or playing animal roles (like the fetish where men and women prance like horses and wear saddles and bits or the fetish that includes getting frisky while wearing a plush animal costume). To each her own enjoyment!

7. GIRL-ON-GIRL FANTASY

The girl-on-girl vision is wildly popular because, for one, it's constantly played out in hot, ravishing style in books and movies, so we've all experienced it in a way. Also, it's easy to imagine the feel of a female's soft, curvy body and how her hair would glide across your skin because we all have the same foxy equipment. And there's no question that a woman will know what makes other women go wild!

8. STARRING IN A NAUGHTY MOVIE

Ever think about being the lead actress in your own sex flick? If it turns you on to be filmed, I recommend you role-play this rather than actually record it, because what if someone else finds it? It's a reality that must be considered. Then again, maybe the danger of discovery is part of the thrill! If you do hit RECORD, proceed with much thought and great caution—and store the video in a secure place.

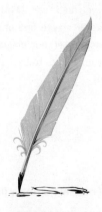

**JOURNALING
EXERCISE**

Part 1: Define What
Fantasies Turn You On

After you're done rating the fantasies, grab your journal and jot down the elements that have stuck with you. You'll then use these notes as the basic ingredients to craft a fully written fantasy story in the next exercise, below. For now, don't worry about award-winning prose; this is an outline only. Include • *Who* (Name the starring players.) • *What* (What story line you fancy—getting it on with a gladiator? The pizza guy? A secret agent? Your hot neighbor?) • *When* (Do you tie your erotic thrills to a certain time of your life, an ancient time, or a future time?) • *Where* (Is your fantasy location a certain room in your house or another house, or is it in a sex club; a wet, dark city street; a sunny beach in Tahiti?) • *How* (How do you see your role playing out: being the aggressor or the one being chased?) • *Overall vibe* (Write down whatever gives your fantasy its thrill factor. Was there a sense of background danger that played into the scenarios you liked most? Or a sense of romance?)

Part 2: Write a *Sexy Story*!

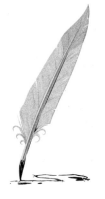

**JOURNALING
EXERCISE**

this journaling exercise, I want you to grab some quiet time in a sexy space (like your newly revamped boudoir!), and write out a fantasy of your own. Think of it like a movie, with a beginning, a middle, and an end. Turn on some tunes, adjust the lights, and put pen to paper. Include plenty of sensual details like touch, smell, feel, and taste. And emotional details, too. How do you feel? Fearful? Trusting? Excited? Aggressive? Devious? Or maybe free of all thoughts except your desire for pleasure? Let your imagination go wherever it wants. This is your chance to have the sex you've always dreamed of!

CONGRATS—YOU'VE GOT FANTASIES!
NOW WHAT?

Enjoy them for your own blissful pleasure, and share them, of course! It's totally fine to keep some fantasies to yourself. (And in some cases, it's prudent to do so. If you fantasized about getting it on with a business partner or your ex, you might want to keep that in the vault.) You can use these to turn yourself on before you have sex with your lover or as you prepare to have a sexy session with yourself.

Your fantasies can be used as terrific verbal foreplay with a lover. Telling someone your fantasy is a huge turn-on, to both your lover and yourself. Whispering a snippet of a fantasy in your lover's ear and seeing how he reacts will tell you how he feels about the subject matter. You could say something like, *The other night, that incredible double-handed move you did made me feel as if I was being serviced by two people. It was so hot; I haven't stopped thinking about it.* And it's okay to be direct, too! Try something like, *This is just a mental fantasy that turns me on—I don't want to actually dress up as a pirate wench and walk the "plank" into our pool—but let me tell you what I've been dreaming about us doing together.*

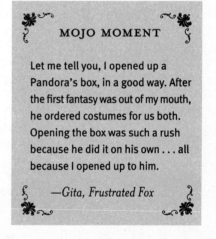

You know your partner, so offer up as much as you think he'll be cool with, then decide how much more you want to reveal. Trust me—most men will join in the banter and will try to draw out *more* details from you . . . They live for the moment when you bust out your vampy side.

For the fantasies you actually want to act out as a couple, you'll need to get your partner onboard, naturally. Bringing the subject up can be done in several manners. *Showing* your fantasy is a simple way to break the ice on a risqué subject. Share erotic magazines, DVDs, porn Web sites, or even conventional

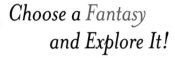

Choose a Fantasy *and Explore It!*

EXERCISE

If you're single, enjoy at least one fantasy-inspired solo session. Part of a couple? Do the same, but include your lover. Replay it in your head and reflect on how you felt before, during, and after. Then pick up your journal and express how it felt.

❤ How did it feel to share your fantasy? Bold? Scary? Empowering?

❤ Did you act out the fantasy word for word? Parts of it? Did it lead you into frisky business?

❤ Did this exercise increase intimacy between you and your lover? Make you laugh? Freak you out? Help you overcome any fears of expressing yourself?

❤ Do you feel that this exercise helped open up new possibilities for pleasure between you and your lover— new possibilities for sexy adventures?

❤ Could exploring your fantasies help deepen your sexual connection moving forward?

❤ Did actively pursuing a fantasy boost your confidence? Why?

❤ Did this give you an idea for an exciting new fantasy? What is it?

books or movies where your fantasies are main plot points (for example, *Threesome* is about—you guessed it—a threesome!), and ask what your partner thinks. You could even play a little game where you each write a few fantasies on index cards or slips of paper, trade them, and then read each other's fantasies. You could then rate the ones you want to try together and set a fantasy date for once a week or month, where you explore a different scenario each time. Definitely tap

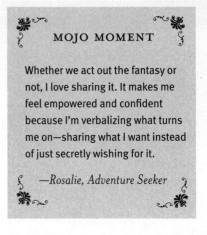

MOJO MOMENT

Whether we act out the fantasy or not, I love sharing it. It makes me feel empowered and confident because I'm verbalizing what turns me on—sharing what I want instead of just secretly wishing for it.

—Rosalie, Adventure Seeker

into the new and improved communication skills that you learned in Chapter 10 and let him know what you want and that you want to get him involved. This gives you a chance to see if he's onboard, and to what extent. Does he want to go all out, for a full role-playing production? Is he comfortable tying you up or spanking you or being spanked himself? This can also be a good opportunity to find out what his fantasies are!

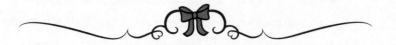

OKAY, ENOUGH INSTRUCTION, ENOUGH THINKING.
ARE YOU READY TO PUT IT ALL INTO ACTION?
I KNOW YOU ARE. IT'S TIME TO FLAUNT IT.

CHAPTER SEVENTEEN

Creating Flirtation

A**T THIS POINT IN THE MOJO MAKEOVER, YOU'RE FLYING HIGH** in your own world of sexiness. Now it's time to get out there and push the envelope a little more with some fun flirting. Flirting—giving attraction and getting attraction—is a natural, healthy, fun part of any sexy self-confident lifestyle. With a little guidance, you'll be an expert in no time.

I define flirting in broad terms. It's not just a tool for picking up a hot specimen at a bar. At its most basic level, it's about giving and getting positive energy, and that, in turn, provides an emotional boost. In some situations, it can have nothing to do with sex or sexiness. Think of a bright-eyed baby who coos at you on line in the grocery store. You start smiling and cooing back and forth. He's flirting with you, and it couldn't be more innocent—he loves the positive energy he gets back. And you do, too.

Of course, flirtiness can have everything to do with sex and sexiness and nailing a hottie. In fact, there are three types of flirting.

You should embrace them as they fit into your life, as part of your Mojo Makeover long after it's completed:

1. FLIRTING TO GIVE AND GET POSITIVITY

You should do this with men, women, kids, and even pets—it's not sexual. It's about reaching out and touching someone . . . spreading a good mood. These can be quick conversations where you sprinkle your energy all over the place. At the gym, complimenting another woman's spinning top because it makes her arms look good is this type of flirtation. So is joking with the UPS guy about his wearing shorts when it's forty degrees out or telling your fave deli owner that he makes the best veggie soup and that you've told all your friends.

You see what I mean? Connecting in a fun way makes you feel good, which supports your mission to feel confident and lit up in your daily life. You're projecting your good feelings onto others, and you'll start to become aware of them when they're being aimed back at you.

2. FLIRTING TO ATTRACT A SEXY BEAST

Of course if you're single, you'll want to shower someone with come-hither flirtiness. The more you practice it (try it on a friend or in the mirror), the readier you'll be when it comes time to lay it on someone you do want to pick up. Having a prop is a great conversation starter *(My puppy seems to like you!)*. So is a cool

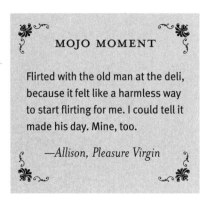

gadget *(OMG, have you seen this crazy app?)* or even a book or crossword puzzle *(Hey, you look like someone who might be able to help me. Do you know a six-letter word for impressionist?)*.

Avoid cliché pickup lines like, *What's your sign?* and opt instead for honest, upfront flirting, like, *Hi, I'm Debbie. You really caught my eye, so I thought I'd come over and say . . . hi.* Then choose some kind of outside topic, person, or object to talk about instead of the typical *What brings you here? What do you do for a living?* types of questions that tend to bore people (you included).

Bring up the new traveling art exhibit in town. Ask him what his opinion is of the band that just got off stage. Ask him whether he's seen the latest YouTube sensation. Or use compliments. Everyone loves to be complimented, but pose them as a question, which will open a conversation like, *You look like an athlete. Do you train for a sport?* Or, *I love your style. Are you an artist?*

3. FLIRTING TO CONNECT WITHIN YOUR RELATIONSHIP

Although I don't think it's done consciously, most women stop flirting once they're in a committed relationship. Who says you can't flirt? I'm married, but I'm not dead! I love the attention my husband showers on me, but that doesn't mean

I don't want to feel desired by others. It's human nature to want that! And it's also human nature for me to desire others—but since I'm in a deeply committed relationship, I know that that's where it stops for me. So, a bit of light flirting fuels my fire, boosts my confidence, and affirms just how sexy I feel, and then I bring *all* that home to my husband.

Don't get me wrong; I'm not flirting with single young men. I'm flirting innocently with a celebrity I see across the room at a restaurant in L.A., or with construction workers outside of buildings on my New York City press trips, or with an acquaintance at a dinner party that I know is fully aware that I'm a happily coupled lady. And on top of that, I'm flirting like *crazy* with my hubbie! I'm giving him light smacks on the bottom when he's fresh out of the shower. I straddle his leg at the office when he's trying to concentrate. I seductively lean over his computer so he gets a good view of my cleavage. I lean in to whisper dirty things in his ear during a business meeting. So I know that he's benefiting from all this flirting, too, in both a direct and indirect way.

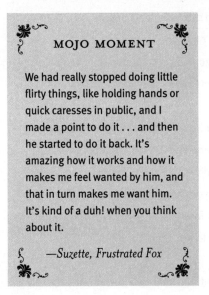

MOJO MOMENT

We had really stopped doing little flirty things, like holding hands or quick caresses in public, and I made a point to do it . . . and then he started to do it back. It's amazing how it works and how it makes me feel wanted by him, and that in turn makes me want him. It's kind of a duh! when you think about it.

—*Suzette, Frustrated Fox*

HOOK A HOTTIE—
FLIRTING TECHNIQUES TO TRY

Body movement is an important facet of flirting to attract someone. Practice these moves in a mirror *and* on a friend to see what feels natural, and then try it out for real. If your object of desire doesn't respond to your flirtatious signals, simply move on—you don't know what's going on in that person's head. Connecting might be the last thing he wants, and that's nothing personal.

💜 **Twirl your hair.** Playing with your hair can be used to attract your target's attention. It's ultrafeminine and a classic symbol of flirtation. While you twirl your hair, remember to expose your kissable neck, adding a trace of your fingers subtly across your skin. Slightly turn your head and face to the side and down a bit, and add a flirtatious, coy glance to the side.

💜 **Hold the gaze.** When you've identified someone you want to flirt with, give him a soft, seductive gaze, and when he catches you looking, hold it for a few seconds, then look away. Then do it again. He'll know you're flirting, and you'll know whether he's interested if he holds your gaze. If he doesn't, move on.

💜 **Add in a lightning-fast wink.** I love a sexy wink; it's a lost art, and admittedly, it can appear stalker-y if done too literally. I recommend doing a soft, not-too-slow, not-too-fast double-eyed blink during your gaze. (So blink, then wink immediately after—got it?) It's a subtle doe-eyed tribute to the classic wink, but without cheesiness.

💜 **Show your curves.** Arching your back presses your sexy bust forward naturally, and your curvy bum back. Try it just ever . . . so . . . slightly when someone is looking at you. It will light up his mind and make you feel super seductive and feminine.

💜 **Bite or lick your lips.** A little nibble on the corner of your mouth or even a tiny lick at the corner of your upper lip is a superb visual reference for your flirting object to see. It will get his wheels turning, imagining what other seductive maneuvers your lips can do. Don't be too obvious or pornographic about this. Just be subtle, subtle, subtle, as if you really are licking something off— imagine there's a dot of cappuccino froth there.

💜 **Cross and uncross your legs.** How memorable is Sharon Stone for her seductive flash in *Basic Instinct*? I'm not suggesting you flash your muff to flirt with the guy across the room, but the simple act of crossing and uncrossing your legs when you're in a skirt or dress is seriously seductive. It emphasizes your gorgeous gams, showcases your feet tucked into high heels, and gives his eye a flash of the arch of your foot, which is quite a classic sexual referent.

💜 **Touch flirtatiously.** If you're already engaged in conversation, casual touches on the arm will let the person you're flirting with know that you're definitely flirting with him.

💜 **Smile!** You're happy to be there, happy to be flirting, happy to be living up to your sexiest self. Happiness is sexy, and happiness is approachable!

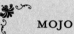

MOJO MOMENT

The more I flirt, the more comfortable I've gotten with the fact that it works! And I'm getting flirted with, too! In practice, a combination of holding a gaze and smiling is definitely an invitation to a conversation opener. When I feel nervous about going to an event alone, I now rely on these standbys.

—Dara, Late Bloomer

 MOJO MEMO:

Flirting for Fun:
How to Keep It Innocent

Now if you're coupled up, you need to make sure you don't cross certain lines, because even if you have the best, most angelic intentions, you might unwittingly send devilish thoughts flaring through another man's head. These tips will help you establish boundaries right off the bat so that it's clear your flirting is meant for fun only.

💜 **SAY YOU'RE TAKEN.** This states very clearly to the person you're flirting with that things are not going to go beyond this fun, frisky conversation. Slip it in within the first few minutes.

If you're asked where you live, reply, *I live in West Hollywood with my boyfriend*. Or, if you're asked, *What do like to do on weekends?* Say, *I train for marathons with my boyfriend*, or, *I've been gardening like crazy. My husband and I are dead set on finally growing our own tomatoes*. You get the idea: find a way to loop your guy in. *Yes, I have been to Las Vegas; my husband and I went last year for our anniversary*.

❤ **NO NUMBER OR E-MAIL EXCHANGES ALLOWED.** That's giving a mixed message to him, and it's taking it too far for you. Unless it's legitimately for business reasons (and it never really is), taking his card is just asking for trouble. If he asks for yours, it's time to end the interaction.

❤ **THERE SHOULD BE NO TOUCHING.** If he touches you, he's into you, and it's time to move on so he can, too.

❤ **CONVERSATIONS SHOULD BE RATED G.** You should *not* talk about sex or fantasies or body part (yours, his, or anyone's). Nothing remotely sexual! That just leads to trouble.

❤ **MAKE SURE YOUR PARTNER IS ONBOARD.** Be considerate of your partner's feelings. Not everyone is secure enough to feel okay if his girlfriend or wife flirts, however innocently. On the flip side, I highly encourage you to have a conversation with your man about the fact that you enjoy a bit of harmless flirting, and that you love to bring it home to *him*. You have to figure out what feels right in your relationship, together.

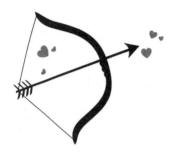

EXERCISE

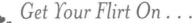

Get Your Flirt On . . .

You can guess what this exercise will be, right? Take one of the above flirting moves and try it out! Don't forget to write about what you did, what reactions you got, and how it affected your Mojo!

Enjoy Your Flirty Groove!

I predict that very soon you're going to notice that you're flashing smiles at strangers and they're smiling back. (And maybe you'll even store one of those strangers in your mental vault to star in your next fantasy!) Your hips are swaying a bit more; you're twirling your hair a little bit when your heartthrob barista steams your milk at Starbucks. There are more double takes being shot your way; you're hearing, *You're beautiful!* as you pass the deli . . . and you like it. You like it because you're in a confident place and you're in charge of your Mojo!

NO QUESTION: YOU'RE FEELING LIT UP FROM ALL THE WORK YOU'VE BEEN DOING IN YOUR MOJO MAKEOVER. YOU'RE MORE ORGASMIC, YOU'RE FEELING FEMININE, SEXY, ALIVE—THE WORLD IS YOUR OYSTER! NEXT UP, I'M GOING TO GIVE YOU A BREAK WITH A CHAPTER THAT FOCUSES ON HOW FAR YOU'VE COME. PUT YOUR FEET UP AND ENJOY IT!

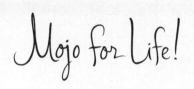

Mojo for Life!

It's the end, and the beginning! You can't finish up without doing some final soul-searching and self-congratulations. You deserve to have everything you've worked for. Let's lock it all down before you strut into a sexy, self-satisfied, and confident sunset.

AS A FINAL SEND-OFF YOU'LL

- ❤ Identify and smooth out any lingering issues with some final exercises and journaling work.

- ❤ Stock your creative arsenal with more racy sex scenarios (because a girl can never have too many ideas!).

- ❤ Touch base with your Mojo Model, how she has evolved and how to keep her going strong.

CHAPTER EIGHTEEN

Taking Inventory

I**T'S TIME TO SLOW DOWN A LITTLE AND REFLECT ON HOW FAR** you've come. This is an easy, all-journaling exploration. Fill your coffee cup or wineglass, light a candle, and find a quiet spot to relax and answer the questions below. The prompts are designed to help you take stock in your Mojo Makeover progress so you can thoroughly appreciate your hard work. Be as detailed as possible and share all your emotions! Remember, there are no wrong answers here, and if there are any tiny wrinkles left, this will be your chance to identify them so you can polish them smooth before your makeover wraps up.

You'll see that I've sprinkled in some snippets of positive self-talk. I want you to say each statement out loud to celebrate yourself before you tackle each section. Then as you write, take every morsel of credit that you can for being such a go-getter during your makeover journey. You deserve it, and you *are* awesome!

1. DESCRIBE YOUR SEXY SELF-CONFIDENCE LEVEL

The seductive,
in-control woman
I am today
has always been inside,
waiting to
come out and play.

1. How has your relationship with yourself changed? Are you experiencing more self-love and less negative body banter?

2. Do you feel more empowered to put yourself and your desires out there?

3. Has your ability to express what you find sexy improved through this process? Has how you feel about yourself improved?

2. JOT DOWN SOME POSITIVE BODYBANTER

Self-consciousness will
no longer drag me down.
I have the tools
to push past it
and never look back.

1. What parts of your body have you become kinder to? Have you fallen in love with a sexy part of yourself that you used to overlook?

2. Are there still parts of yourself that you're beating up? What's holding you back from fully embracing them and showering them with sexy self-love?

3. Can you step in front of the mirror, touch a part you're still down on, and just switch up your feelings right now? Kick that annoying inner critic to the curb—you have no need for her anymore!

3. CHALLENGE YOURSELF
TO COMMUNICATE

Opening up about what I desire has made me more satisfied in all aspects of my life.

1. How would you describe the changes that have occurred in your ability to communicate about sex and your desires?

2. With your new communication skills, have you been able to get more of what you want by expressing yourself?

3. Are there desires you still feel uncomfortable expressing? Why? How might you use what you've learned to embrace this?

4. GIVE YOURSELF PERMISSION
TO FULLY ENJOY YOUR SEXUALITY

Permission is self-worth. I will never forget it.

1. Before the makeover, what were the obstacles that kept you from giving yourself permission to bring your Mojo into the forefront of your life?

2. Where in the makeover did you experience a breakthrough with this?

3. Knowing what you know now, what would you say to your former self to give her permission to explore her seductive side?

5. THINK SEXY THOUGHTS
EVERY DAY

Opening my mind to sexy opportunities has opened my eyes to many pleasures in my life.

1. Do you feel like you have more sex "on the brain" now that the makeover is almost complete?

2. Which exercise or exercises really flipped on the switch that made you "see" sex all around your daily life?

3. What has this influenced the most? Your overall sexy self-confidence? Your desire for more sex? Has it pushed you to carry yourself differently out in the world? Or has it influenced something else?

6. EXPRESS YOUR SELF-LOVE BY
CLAIMING WHAT YOU DESERVE

I've created my own personal sexy revolution and have come out the other side fulfilled and excited to embrace a sexier lifestyle.

1. What role did self-love play in your life before the Mojo Makeover?

2. What is its role today—now that you've been practicing self-love techniques?

3. Which exercises ignited your understanding of what self-love is? Mirror dancing? Positive affirmations during your beauty and body routine? Satisfying yourself during the Big 5-O program?

7. ACKNOWLEDGE YOUR LUST FOR LIFE!

Nurturing desire
makes all parts of my life
more thrilling.
It's a gift I give to myself.

1. Have you found that creating seductive sanctuaries—a welcoming bedroom, a closet you love browsing through, a yummy bath ritual—have influenced the way you care for yourself?

2. Did tackling risqué explorations (like fantasies, sexy talk, or flirting) give you a solid sense of owning your desire? Why?

FINISHED?

By now your confidence must be swelling (and yes, your hand may be cramping). Your journal is becoming a keepsake that you will love to touch back on for fun and for frisky ideas, and to inspire yourself when you need a reminder that you possess the desire and drive to make a positive change in your life. You *can* do the hard work and face tough (as well as red-hot, kinky, sexy) challenges and succeed wildly! The evidence is there on every one of your pages. I'm so proud of you!

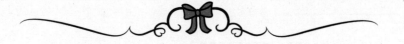

IF YOU FIND THAT YOU'VE GOT A FEW CRINKLES
IN YOUR PROGRAM, DON'T WORRY.
THE NEXT CHAPTER, YOUR SECOND-TO-LAST,
IS YOUR FINAL DIAGNOSTIC TUNE-UP TO ENSURE
THAT ALL YOUR MOJO ENGINES ARE RUNNING
AT FULL CAPACITY. EVEN IF YOU'RE AT
FULL THROTTLE RIGHT NOW, YOU'LL STILL PICK UP
SOME NEW TRICKS—I'VE SAVED SOME OF THE
JUICIEST ONES FOR THE END!

CHAPTER NINETEEN

Even More Sexy Scenarios for Now (or Later)

READY FOR SEX, SEX, AND MORE SEX? I'VE CREATED A ROSTER of erotic experiences below. They're meant to inspire real dates that you can enjoy (with yourself or a lover) to keep your Mojo strong. With each, I've painted a picture that includes the tools, frame of mind, conversations, and signature moves to create the ultimate sexy experience. You can follow any of them step-by-step for the utmost confidence.

There are fifteen scenarios below. Find the ones that speak to you, and by all means, if you feel inspired to change them up—go for it! In fact, as this week's exercise, I want you to experience two of them! And of course, as with all of your adventures thus far, don't forget the condoms—safe is sexy, baby!

MOJO MOMENT

I've never been one to do solo sessions. But starting with an
adventure seemed like a good way to try it, like I was in a
movie. I had never gone to a bar by myself. Just knowing my
purpose made it feel illicit and actually a turn-on! I had a lot of
fun alone at home later, and it inspired me to start solo sessions.
I guess I needed that kick-start!

—*Tessa, Late Bloomer*

ACCESSORIES

Plumping lip gloss
Cream rouge
Seductive body cream
High heels
Sexy panties
Your two favorite toys
Lubricant

1. SEXY SOLO DATE

Take yourself out for a cocktail and a light dinner at a
local bar (one you're already familiar with, where you
feel safe). First, dress to impress . . . yourself! Start
with some seductive beauty rituals (gloss your lips;
rouge your cheeks; butter up your bod with a scented
cream). Adorn yourself with a pair of pretty undies, a
hot outfit, and a sexy pair of heels, and venture out
feeling lit up. Saunter up to the bar, order a sexy

cocktail and a light bite. As you sip, think about the amazing orgasm you're going
to give yourself when you get home. Imagine what the bartender (or other
spotted object of desire) looks like with his clothes off. Indulge in every morsel
of food you're eating, teasing up your taste buds.

Since this is a solo date, don't engage in too much conversation with others—
unless you're single and looking for a date! Then head home, hit the bedroom,

and dim the lights. Turn on music, and do the Slow Walk to your bed. Twist and Dip down to your bedside drawer, where you've left not one but two of your favorite sex toys.

Start with one toy over your panties. Breathing slowly, revel in all your sexiness, undulate on the bed with desire for yourself. When you're ready to take off your panties, do so by teasing yourself, as a lover would. Pull one corner down, then back up, writhing your hips around, until your panties are by your knees. You can arch your back, raise your legs, and kick them off. As the desire and intensity build, pull back. Tease yourself. Draw this out! Build up again, and as you're getting closer to orgasm, reach for your second toy.

If you've been working your C-Spot, add the second toy for V-Spot pleasure, or tempt your A-Spot—whatever is going to give you the biggest, most explosive orgasm possible! For an added element of sexiness, position yourself in front of your mirror and watch yourself experience the pure satisfaction of your orgasm. *Damn,* don't you feel sexy?

ACCESSORIES

Easy-access clothing, like skirts and crotchless panties

A disposable vibrating couples ring

Discreet vibrator, like a lipstick shape

2. HOT NEW–RELATIONSHIP SEX

(Note: You can do this when you're really in a new relationship or if you're already coupled up for years— simply act this out as a fantasy, recalling the hot, hot heat you had when you first met.)

You and your new lover are hot and frisky, doing it every day, or at least four to five times a week, and the energy behind your sex is intense, frenzied, desirous,

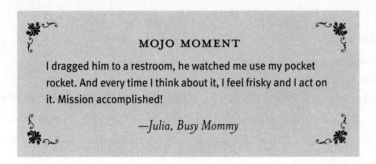

> **MOJO MOMENT**
>
> I dragged him to a restroom, he watched me use my pocket rocket. And every time I think about it, I feel frisky and I act on it. Mission accomplished!
>
> —*Julia, Busy Mommy*

insatiable, and adventurous. Those frisky feelings aren't hitting you just when you're snuggled up at his apartment but everywhere, all the time. Great! It's your opportunity to take it outdoors (and anywhere else you happen to be). Park the car in a secluded spot, jump in the backseat, and grind your clothed bodies together like teenagers until you tear them off; then rock the car back and forth with your in-sync thrusting. Or find a park late at night, and let him give you oral pleasure on the swing set, through your crotchless panties. Or, if you bring him home to meet your parents, do it in your teenage bed or in the garage after everyone else is asleep. Even racier, drag him into a private bathroom at a restaurant where you've met up with friends for dinner. Pleasure yourself while he watches, and when you both return to the table, he'll have that vision locked in his mind.

Your options here are limitless. Why not add in accessories like a pocket vibrator, minipackets of lubricant, or disposable vibrating couples rings, which are packaged with some intimacy kits? This is the time in your relationship when anything goes and the frequency is driven by mad desire. Use it wisely. Live out the adventure!

ACCESSORIES

Lubricant (lots)

A-Spot vibrator

C-Spot vibrator

3. TAKING THINGS FURTHER

You've been having hot sex with your boyfriend (or husband) for several months, and have a strong sense of intimacy and trust. If you're curious about A-Spot sex, why not explore it now?

First, you'll need to be fully relaxed and committed to taking the experience slowly. Let him pamper you with an all-over sensual massage—drizzling oil all over your breasts, caressing and rubbing your cheeks and thighs, making lovely large circles upward, toward your lower back. You'll be totally turned on, open to a whole new world of pleasure possibilities, and perhaps a little nervous. Remember to breathe and relax—and of course, to use copious amounts of lubricant every step of the way. Let him massage your A-Spot first, then slide in a finger, and then a toy—try to contain your orgasm until the big moment: his shaft (also coated with lots of lubricant).

As a beginner, start by positioning yourself on top first, where you'll have the most control. Just breathe through the initial sensation of insertion and relax.

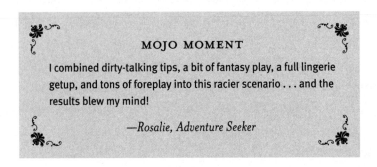

MOJO MOMENT

I combined dirty-talking tips, a bit of fantasy play, a full lingerie getup, and tons of foreplay into this racier scenario . . . and the results blew my mind!

—*Rosalie, Adventure Seeker*

Add in a C-Spot vibrator to move toward an orgasm, but don't go racing toward any kind of thrusting! Just get used to the feeling and then start to move your body against him in a way that feels right to you. Anytime you need to, add more lubricant! This is a great opportunity to use your dirty-talk skills because this kind of sex carries a taboo, a certain naughtiness. It makes you feel a bit wanton and wild. You're in the big girls' club now, baby. So use your vocal cords; move your hips; tell him how dirty he is; cry out with abandon!

ACCESSORIES

Costume

Panties

Toys

Lubricant, massage oil, or other romantic treats

Food

Creativity

4. REIGNITE YOUR RELATIONSHIP WITH A TEN-DAY SEX MARATHON

It happens to all married and long-term couples. A week goes by without sex. Then, *Wait, has it been ten days? Oh no . . . it's been two weeks!* Having a sex marathon—committing to several days in a row of getting it on—will help you both reclaim your enthusiasm and get back in the swing of things. Look at a calendar together and choose a reasonable stretch of time (ten days, not thirty).

Prepare for it by thinking through what you can wear and toys and other props (like foods, a fire in the fireplace) that will keep things fresh. Make a mental list of locations in the house where you can do it: the bedroom, living room, guest room, patio, kitchen, bathroom, garage! Try different times of the day and different kinds of action for variety. Morning quickies, midday baths with waterproof toys, midnight oral—or grab him for a go before he heads for the gym. Look back to Chapter 16 and try out a new fantasy scenario. Focus on talking dirty for one session, then focus another on all the kissing techniques, sensual foods, or other foreplay scenarios you've learned. Bring in sexy panties, a blindfold, a couples toy, even a costume. The frequency will force you to seek variety, and the combination of lots of different kinds of sex will remind you how much pleasure you and your lover can bring to each other!

ACCESSORIES

Massage oil

Pleasure sleeve
(optional)

Lubricant

5. AWFUL-SEX INTERVENTION

All couples become out of sync at some point or another. He's got high stress levels from work. She's anxious about something, too. Whatever the causes, the result is never fun—you end up having distracted, disconnected, and frustratingly Awful Sex. You know what I mean: It's taking you an hour to come, or you just give up. You're really craving penetration, but he loses his erection or blasts off within thirty seconds. You lay there thinking, *This kind of sucks*.

But it's not a disaster. It's most likely a temporary setback, and you *have* to talk about it. Breeze through Chapter 10 to brush up on your communication skills. Snuggle up and have a chat about what's been happening and how you both can bring the magic back.

Then get back in the saddle. Start with lots of intimate kissing, massaging, and just being together. If he lost his erection the last time, he's going to feel pressure—and performance anxiety—and that can lead to another downer. So build the passion slowly. Agree that this time isn't about reaching orgasm; it's

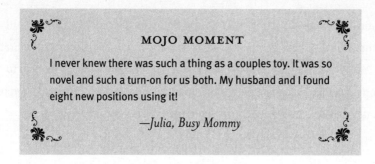

MOJO MOMENT

I never knew there was such a thing as a couples toy. It was so novel and such a turn-on for us both. My husband and I found eight new positions using it!

—*Julia, Busy Mommy*

about reconnecting and feeling close. Sometimes a guy can use some extra help. Next time you could make a session all about his pleasure, starting with a massage and head-to-toe kisses. Try a pleasure sleeve to stroke his member with different sensations than the norm, and add in plenty of oral. If he senses that you're enjoying him, as opposed to expecting something from him, he's more likely to relax and, in turn, get his groove back. And he can do the same for you, with an all-you night, as you two reclaim your passion.

6. FRISKY GETAWAY SEX

ACCESSORIES

Vibrating panties

Sneak away to a cheap motel for a night! Surprise your guy the first time out, and then turn it into a regular thing. After you two check in, lock yourself in the bathroom and slide into a pair of vibrating panties, then pull on your sexiest jeans over them. Tell your guy you want to hit up the local burger joint for dinner. Once there, slide the panties' remote control across the table. If he wonders what it is, press ON and take his hand to your inner thigh; he'll feel the vibrations and immediately want to play.

As you enjoy your beers and frisky conversation, he'll scroll through the settings on the remote, taking you for a wild ride of pulsing, surging, escalating, vibrating fun. You'll need to work on keeping a straight face, while he won't be able to stand up without exposing his desire. See how long you two can take it before you race back to the hotel and start your naughty little night away.

ACCESSORIES

Butterfly-style strap-on vibrator

Couples vibrator

Waterproof toy for the shower

Lubricant

7. BUSY MOMMY SEX

This is about grabbing opportunities on the fly and shagging fast and crazy. Frantic sex: hot, fresh, and seriously satisfying. The quickest way to do that is by building your sex toy collection. Try a butterfly strap-on vibrator so you can be intensely stimulated as you give your man an oral treat. Or pick up a mind-blowing couples toy so you can ride your man and a multifunction C-Spot vibrator at the same time. Lube can get both of your bodies worked up faster, and you can try solo sessions next to each other (because you each know how to get yourself off best). There's absolutely nothing wrong with a pull-your-jeans-down, fun-in-the-laundry-room quickie or jumping into the shower together for sex (with a waterproof toy!) and shampoos at once. You don't want your entire sex life to be fast and furious, but taking advantage of those moments can add a lusty thrill—and, of course, the more Os in your world, the better!

ACCESSORIES

Sexy bubble bath

Waterproof toy

Fun food to share,
like cheese,
desserts, wine

Board or card games

Sexy massage oil

8. THE RUT BUSTER

In a sex rut? It happens, especially when couples do their own thing night after night. If you both work or the kids are a handful, night becomes the only "me time" either of you has and it's natural to want to chill out. But often that means one of you goes online and the other watches TV, or he does his hobby while you read a book. You need some romance, some together time—a date!

Even if you can't leave the house (because of the kids or the budget or both) devote one hour a week to a special date. Dress to impress yourself and each other and have a miniparty. (Be sure to do some flirting!) This could be a cheese tasting for two, wine and cake that you made for this night, or a game you used to love to play together. (Scrabble, Jenga, poker—every couple has a game.) You could cozy up in a bubble bath that's completed by a sexy setup—meaning the

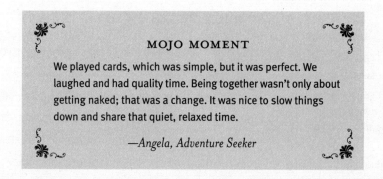

MOJO MOMENT

We played cards, which was simple, but it was perfect. We laughed and had quality time. Being together wasn't only about getting naked; that was a change. It was nice to slow things down and share that quiet, relaxed time.

—*Angela, Adventure Seeker*

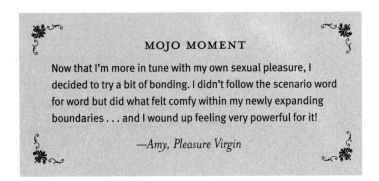

MOJO MOMENT

Now that I'm more in tune with my own sexual pleasure, I decided to try a bit of bonding. I didn't follow the scenario word for word but did what felt comfy within my newly expanding boundaries . . . and I wound up feeling very powerful for it!

—*Amy, Pleasure Virgin*

candles, the special bubble bath, a purring massage mitt, or a waterproof toy. His and hers massage nights would be a sweet treat.

Date nights can be as simple as these. What's important is treating it like a date and making it happen. That connecting time will help ignite intimacy—think of it as the sex before the sex—and in feeling more connected, you'll want to connect physically.

ACCESSORIES

Bonding tape
(or silk ties or scarves)

Some form of
dominatrix wand
(a spanker, whipper, etc.)

Ice cubes

Vibrating couples ring

9. THE BIG BONDING TEASE

You're in a frisky mood and you feel like tying up your man. Time to try bonding. Create a dominatrix-inspired outfit, like a black corset with high-heeled thigh-high boots, that'll get his mind going wild. Or wrap bonding tape around your bust line to create a sexy bandeau top and around your hips for a racy miniskirt, then let your lover unwind you. Use the tape to tie his wrists and ankles to the bedposts. Tonight, you'll get to be in control of your lover's pleasure. Tease and delight him with kisses, caresses, ice cubes, and more until he's on the brink; then back off, build him up again, then back off again. Add in other, bonding-type accessories like a spanker or a whipper made of rubber strands, and alternate using soft strokes with friskier taps to stimulate the skin. Use dirty talk and tell him he's been a *very bad boy* and he's going to pay for it by nailing you silly. Let him watch you touch yourself; not being able to touch you will drive him crazy. Straddle his face, then pull away, just out of his mouth's reach, then come back and lose yourself in oral pleasure. When you're ready, hop on his shaft and ride him till you reach orgasm (use your vibrating couples ring for extra C-Spot stimulation if you like). Alternatively, play the submissive role and let him tie you up and build your excitement till you can't stand the tease!

10. SEXY VIDEO SHOOT

ACCESSORIES

A camera operator
(i.e., your lover or
your computer)

Decadent shimmering
body cream

A sexy outfit: corset,
garters—the works

A sex toy (optional)

Sexy stripping tunes

Lots of moxie

This can be something you do together (and then perhaps even view as a warm-up for your solo sessions), or you can create it with your computer's built-in video camera as a surprise to your lover, to watch together. It can be soft and sexy or extra raunchy. Just be careful with what you do with the video. I can't stress that enough! If you're a first timer, you'll probably feel nervous, which usually means lots of movement. The key is to have enough to do so you don't feel stupid a few minutes into it. So why not make a stripper film? It will give your body plenty to do, and you'll have a clear beginning and end point.

Choose a space in your home where you have room to move. Then shower and slather on a rich shimmering body cream so your skin feels and looks extra succulent, and dress in a super sexy lingerie outfit—garters, a boa, heels—long gloves are a fun thing to strip off. Play some sensual tunes and wriggle slowly to the music, dance using the Twist and Dip move, then slowly peel your outfit off piece by piece, stroking your body with your fingers. Close your eyes and get into it. If you really want to go for broke, include a vibrator and lightly trace it over your neck, nipples, abdomen. You can end it here with a flirty wink and a fade-out. Or, stimulate yourself to an O. It will be super sexy without it, but there's no reason to stop, and it will be quite a sweet ending indeed.

11. THE ALMOST THREESOME

ACCESSORIES

Blindfold

Chocolate body fondue

Feathers or spanker

Lubricant

You read about the threesome fantasy in Chapter 16, but what about when it comes to actually fulfilling the fantasy? If you're into it, go for the real thing. However, I must caution, I do not recommend it, as I've seen it ruin the trust and intimacy couples have built within their relationships. That said, you two could still fulfill the desire for a triple play if you use your imaginations.

If you want it to be about him and two women, blindfold him and play both female roles. First talk through the fantasy with each other (it will get you both

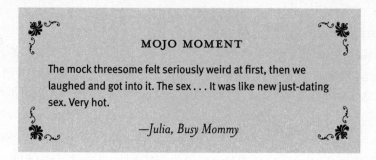

MOJO MOMENT

The mock threesome felt seriously weird at first, then we laughed and got into it. The sex . . . It was like new just-dating sex. Very hot.

—Julia, Busy Mommy

excited and will create a script that you'll both enjoy). Say hello as yourself, and then introduce the "other woman" in the room. Create a second bedroom persona who'll do the things he desires that you're not all that into. Switch up your voice a little bit; touch him in a different way . . . just unleash her on him. Add in sensations you normally wouldn't—like feathers on his skin, light spanking or scratching, or drizzling warm chocolate body fondue all over his shaft and lapping it up. Then, switch back to yourself. Ask him what he thinks of your new partner. Does he like the way she . . . ? What does he want her to do? This may feel strange at first, but practice makes perfect, and remember the goal is to fulfill a fantasy. He's blindfolded, so don't worry about feeling silly. Just throw yourself into it.

Now, if you want to experience another man in your threesome fantasy, purchase a second "shaft" to be in the room. There are unlimited options of gorgeous silicone dildos for you, in all different shapes, sizes, and colors, including *very* realistic male members. Many even have suction-cup bases that'll stick to a headboard so that you can ride it as if it were truly another man. Lube up and hop on for a racy ride!

ACCESSORIES

Two phones
Your favorite sex toy
Lubricant

12. PHONE SEX

He's on a business trip and misses your body. Or, you haven't moved in together and want to keep it hot on the nights you stay at your own pad. You can use phone sex even as a way to spice things up while you're both *in* the same house. Just use your cell from another room.

Create an intensely hot, dirty phone sex encounter, telling him what you want to do to him; how you want to be ravished; how you're touching yourself with a big, hot sex toy; how your knickers are moist from all this phone seduction. If you need ideas in advance, review Chapter 13 for some dirty-talk tips or call a phone sex hotline to get some tips from the pros! Then either invite him to meet you in the bedroom (or some other destination in the house) to bring this phone seduction to a climax, literally, or each of you can bring yourself to orgasm on the phone, in separate rooms. That will add intense anticipation and sexual tension, and he'll probably meet you upstairs in about ten minutes for another go-round. (Just think, you could tally two Os on one day as part of your Big 5-O program!)

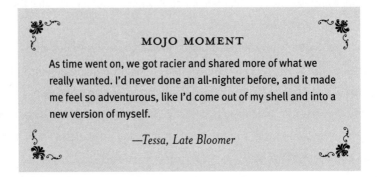

MOJO MOMENT

As time went on, we got racier and shared more of what we really wanted. I'd never done an all-nighter before, and it made me feel so adventurous, like I'd come out of my shell and into a new version of myself.

—*Tessa, Late Bloomer*

ACCESSORIES

Tasty lubricant

Massage candle

Blindfold (or silk scarf
or his neck tie)

Feather body tickler

Leather spanker

Vibrating couples ring

Crotchless panties

13. THE ALL-NIGHT SEDUCTION

Stay up and go at it all night. This is like the sex marathon all jammed into one night. You'll need to invent lots of different vignettes to keep it fresh and frisky for the hours ahead. Think *orgasms solely through oral* (use a delicious kissable lubricant). Enact the classic hot-wax fantasy while blindfolded (use a skin-friendly massage-oil candle so you don't get burned). Bring out a feather tickler and tease him, or use a spanker and give him a dose of loving discipline.

Take a quick nap, then wake your lover up by ducking under the sheets for some kisses on the inner thigh. Move on to make passionate, connected love—classic missionary style, with an added bonus of a vibrating couples ring. Trace ice cubes down each other's bodies while you're in a steamy, hot shower—the hot and cold sensations will be exciting (and so will the sex, pressed up against the shower wall). Cook an early breakfast in his oversize T-shirt and a pair of crotchless knickers so that you're ready to go again right after refueling.

ACCESSORIES

Laptop to play porn

Sexy skivvies

Any toys, lubricants,
and lotions you desire

14. PORN SUNDAY

I hope you've bookmarked some of your favorite porn clips—whether they're soft girl-on-girl scenes with lots of kissing, erotic clips of couples making intensely passionate love, or even raunchier scenes that you found turned you on (against what your good-girl conscience told you should turn you on). Now, it's time to share your newfound affection for visual stimulation with your lover.

One lazy Sunday afternoon, throw on a sexy pair of panties and bra, and invite him into bed for a special experience together, letting him know you'd like to watch some *erotic footage* together. *You mean . . . porn?* he'll ask. To which you will reply, *Yes, darling. Porn!* He'll not only be aroused by the opportunity to watch porn with you, but intrigued and pleasantly surprised that you have favorite clips! (I'm a fan of Youporn.com, a great free site.)

Take control and choose the clip that turns you on the most. (Allow him a turn to choose a clip afterward, if you like.) Try keeping your hands to yourselves for the first few minutes of it, until you simply must reach out and jump each other. Or have a session where you watch an erotic clip and simultaneously self-satisfy, turning your eyes toward each other, then back to the screen, then back again. If it all goes well and you want to repeat it, declare each Sunday "Porn Day." That way, every week when it rolls around, you know you're in for a sexy encounter filled with visual and aural (and, hopefully, oral) stimulation together.

15. PICKING UP A "STRANGER"

ACCESSORIES

Sexy skivvies
Body candle
Whipper

This is where you go out and act as though you and your partner don't know each other. You can take this in so many directions and extend the night as long as you want. Wear a sexy bra and undies (think ones with side tie-ribbons that can be removed with a flick of the wrist later on) and an easy-access skirt or dress. Start at a noisy bar or music club.

Arrive in separate cars or at least park far from the entrance and each take a walk so you can arrive separately and mingle.

Then flirt. (Deploy the tricks from Chapter 17 for picking up a hottie, page 216—use them on your guy and do some innocent flirting with people around you, just as you would if you were a singleton.) Build up the contact with your man slowly, from catching his eyes across the room to sending him a drink, then move closer. Touch his arm. Take on another persona if you each like that— maybe you're a flight attendant on a layover (ha-ha) and he's your favorite hunky actor. You can make this about hot rough sex in the bathroom or alley or take him home to your pad and go nuts on each other using daring toys like fringy whips or hot wax. Try it whenever the opportunity strikes. Pick up each other at a wedding reception or the company picnic.

Finish reading them all? I hope you're formulating when and how you're going to pull off your fave scenarios already. Remember—this week's assignment is to try your favorite two, but this list should keep you getting busy for some time. And there should be plenty of room in your journal for you to keep adding to this list with some of your own ideas and fantasies and accessories. Anytime you hear about a sexy scenario or watch a movie with a great sex scene—jot it down! Keep the creativity flowing for your Mojo's sake!

BELIEVE IT OR NOT, YOUR MAKEOVER IS COMING
TO A CLOSE—THE FINAL CHAPTER IS COMING UP
NEXT. YOU'LL LOOK BACK AND SEE HOW FAR
YOU (AND YOUR MOJO MODEL) HAVE COME
AND WHERE YOU CAN GO FROM HERE. I'VE GOT
PLENTY OF IDEAS FOR HOW TO KEEP YOUR SEXY SELF-
CONFIDENCE ALIVE AND KICKING!

CHAPTER TWENTY

Mojo Model Roundup

I T'S TIME TO SAY GOOD-BYE TO THE MOJO MODEL YOU IDENTIFIED with four weeks ago, and hello to what's next. There's no question, you've shed the Mojo malfunctions that once held you back—but no longer. Still, the work continues! I'm giving you a final cheat sheet of where to keep sharpening and evolving.

Find your former self—your original Mojo Model—take in what I have to say, and keep cultivating that inner vixen!

THE PLEASURE VIRGIN

I know you were especially touched by the exercises that sharpened your focus on what sexy means to *you*, and not just what you think is sexy to a guy. Learning to love yourself and how to appreciate everything you have to offer is a powerful confidence tool, and I want you to continue to work hard to strengthen what you've started. It's important to be in tune with yourself, to appreciate yourself, and to want to feel amazing and confident. As you move ahead, push yourself to explore and bring new options into your sexy lifestyle—reread the fantasies and sexy scenarios in this book and work your way through the list in your own way. You have a great momentum going now . . . Use it to your fullest, juiciest advantage!

THE ADVENTURE SEEKER

You are a showgirl, you love to perform and to express your sexuality in front of others, so sharing your sexy thoughts and trying hot new adventures was easier for you than for other Models. Still, I hope you learned that it's possible for wild sex to become the norm, and not as exciting as it should be (yes, even you can get into a rut) and that you've soaked in some new tricks and treats. Your real challenges in this makeover were the exercises that focused on intimacy—especially connecting to the real, special you. Keep on talking dirty to yourself and to your lover. That exercise works a different set of "sex tools" than you're used to— meaning your verbal skills. Use them regularly so that you continue to build your capacity for emotional intimacy, not just a physical one, with yourself and others.

THE BUSY MOMMY

Self-worship has helped you accept your body and your position in the hierarchy of your busy life. You matter; you deserve; you're so worth it. Keep up with your bath and beauty rituals, your mirror dancing, dressing sexy, and for heaven's sake, do spend the extra few bucks on the lotion with the makes-you-happy scent! Don't slip back into a distant last place on your priority list. And don't get comfortable where you are right now, either—keep kicking your Mojo up a notch and then another notch and then another. Do it by choosing at least one exercise a week that's strictly about keeping your Mojo in high gear. In addition to this, I want you to do at least one activity a week that keeps you and your lover connected—go back to Chapter 16, on fantasies, and Chapter 12, on sexy accessories, for inspiration.

THE FRUSTRATED FOX

No doubt, five orgasms a week has made you a lot less frustrated, with yourself and your lover! You've added some sexy accessories along the way, and that gave you the variety and excitement you may have been lacking and longing for. The Foreplay Challenge should have shaken up your routine and ignited a spark in your relationship; keep at it—try new things! Make a pact with your partner to be equal, active, alive participants in foreplay sessions, to cut loose and not bring any grudges into the bed. Promise each other that you'll be open, fun, and silly. Get frisky at a movie theater; make out in public; show up unannounced at his doorstep or office wearing a trench coat over lingerie; send teasing texts. You each need to keep the variety (and honesty about what you want) going, and you can!

THE LATE BLOOMER

Clearing out the family photos and putting away some of your girlish trinkets has made your bedroom feel sexier, and this exercise probably had the greatest impact on you, of all the Models. It truly symbolized the leap from the *girl who wants* to *the girl who gets what she wants*. It gave you the mental space to think about inviting a lover over and exploring the possibility of finding the love and sex you deserve. Stay busy—mingle, flirt! And if you're single, I encourage you to have lots of fun being one. Look for a social group or a great dating service; don't let the challenge of a bar scene hinder your growth. You've finally bloomed, so go show off that gorgeous flower for everyone to see. Remember, if you put out the message that you are a confident, sexy woman, that is how the world will see you. Now, go get what you want!

YOU'RE ALL LIVING PROOF THAT POSITIVE CHANGES ARE POSSIBLE—THAT YOU JUST NEED TO TAKE ACTION AND MAKE THINGS HAPPEN. IF YOU CAN IDENTIFY PROBLEMS, EVALUATE THEM, STRATEGIZE, AND EXECUTE A GAME PLAN TO CORRECT THE ISSUES, YOU CAN GET TO A PLACE YOU WANT TO BE, AND KNOWING YOU SHOULD ALWAYS BE ON TOP IS KEY TO ENJOYING YOURSELF AND FULFILLING YOUR SEXUAL AND EMOTIONAL NEEDS TO THE FULLEST EXTENT. WAY TO GO!

CHAPTER TWENTY-ONE

You Did It!
Now Keep That Mojo Flowing!

THIS WHOLE PROCESS HAS BEEN ABOUT GIVING YOURSELF permission to discover, develop, and then express your sexiest self. It wasn't to make you into someone you're not or get you to conform to someone else's vision of "sexy." This was *your* journey to find your inner vixen and let her come out and play. Maybe she's been in hiding for years, or maybe you didn't even know she was there. You may have had to let go of old hang-ups, release preconceived notions about deserving satisfaction, or toss out the useless behaviors that made you feel less beautiful, less sexy, less confident than you truly are.

Now that you're back in the saddle and your sexy self-confidence is at an all-time high, I want to keep you there. I also want you to share your knowledge with all your friends! These exercises will ensure that you have everything you need to keep your Mojo burning bright enough for you and those around you, too!

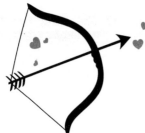
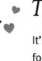

EXERCISE

The *"After"* Photo Session

It's time to take more self-portraits! You'll do the same four shots you snapped for your "before" photo session in the beginning of the book. But now, you're going to see a totally different woman in each image.

♥ PHOTO 1 Running a daily errand

Take a self-portrait before you head out to your Saturday errands. See the difference from your earlier pictures? It's not just what you're wearing or the extra care you've devoted to your beauty prep—though I know your personal style has a friskier come-hither feel now—it's your posture and the confident cock of your head, your coy smile, and a devilish twinkle in your eye that's ready to take on, and take in, the sexiness that's waiting for you.

♥ PHOTO 2 Prepped for a night out

Snap yourself in full-on going out mode. Is that a higher heel than you dared to wear before this journey started? Some more cleavage than you sported four weeks ago? You pull it off *oh so* well, you foxy thing! There's no question that you're up for a wild ride and you're poised to call the shots, whether you're heading out solo or with a lover. The night is yours for the taking. Own it!

♥ PHOTO 3 You at your sexiest

Capture a photo of yourself as undressed as you dare in a setting that makes you feel full of sensuality. Push it to the brink of your comfort, which might mean taking a photo in a low-cut top with a push-up bra that displays sexy cleavage; wearing a camisole and boy shorts with a feather boa; or something more wicked, like full-on

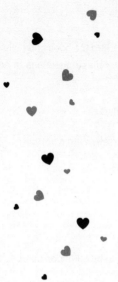

sexy lingerie with garters and heels, nude in a bubble bath, or wrapped in a sheet worshipping and waving your fave new toy at the lens. Go for what really represents the new you. It's for your eyes only!

♥ PHOTO 4　Post-O!

Snap a headshot right after a tantalizing, hot, lusty, mind-blowing orgasm. You don't need to make this a nude photo, and no one who might just happen upon it will know what it's about. Only you will know the pleasure you just experienced when you look back on your rosy, delight-filled face, relaxed posture, and sexy tumbled hair.

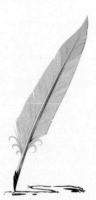

The *"After"* Mojo Makeover Journaling Session

JOURNALING EXERCISE

I want you to think back on the amazing things you've completed that four weeks ago, you never thought you would want to do, could do, or *dare* to do! Anytime we can reflect on how we've tried something new or did something for ourselves or worked really hard to find a solution for something, it gives us a sense of empowerment and ownership over our lives and how we live them. You are in full control of your own sexuality now, and your confidence is soaring!

This exercise is about checking yourself over and taking credit for your new sexy swagger. And if it's not as sexy as you'd like, this activity will help you to pinpoint the areas that still need a bit of tuning up. You can then go back into the book and review, and even retry, the exercises you still need to master. Answer these questions to see where you stand.

- 💜 What were your favorite moments during the makeover? Why?

- 💜 How has the makeover affected your relationship with yourself? With a partner?

- 💜 What differences have you seen in your home life? At work?

- 💜 Do you enjoy talking more about sex?

- 💜 Do you see sex as part of your daily lifestyle now?

- 💜 Are you talking about sex with your friends? Do they seem to be taking on some of your newfound confidence and openness?

- 💜 What fantasies did you bring to life? Which was your favorite?

- 💜 Have your orgasms improved?

- 💜 What sexy scenarios turned you on and delivered?

- 💜 Did any exercises flop? What will it take for you to master them?

- 💜 What other explorations do you see in your near future?

MOJO MAINTENANCE CHECKLIST

Hitting a goal is awesome. Staying there is even sweeter. It's very easy to go coasting on your sexy high, thinking it's going to last forever. But anything that's worth anything requires some TLC. You don't want to wind up back where you started again, only to repeat your bad patterns, get into a slump, or go back to trying things that weren't working in the first place. These suggestions will help keep it in line so your star power doesn't wane.

✓ Schedule Mojo moments into your life

Penciling in hot time may not seem very hot, but for many busy women, it's the only way to ensure they hit their mark, and that's important. When you're ultrabusy, variety can take a backseat because you're not thinking ahead about how to make the most of the time. So use your favorite makeover activities to inspire fun for every date.

♥ If you loved mirror dancing, make every Wednesday night your night to dance and create a sexy solo session.

♥ If flirting and fantasizing struck a chord, Thursday night becomes bar night with the girls. Have a fantasy-inspired sexy solo session before you hit the town, and let that be your sexy inner secret as you flirt the night away.

♥ Did you enjoy acting out different sexy scenarios? Make a pact with your lover that once a week you'll try a totally new theme. Set an e-mail reminder that goes to you and your partner the day before so you can start setting the scene in your minds.

♥ If toys and props made you see stars, schedule in sessions that are solely about accessorized arousal. It will take some thought, which is a good thing because it will keep your busy mind in the saucy moment.

✓ *Keep acting on impulses*

You learned early on in this makeover that ignoring everyday turn-ons, like a sexy scene on TV, a guy you flirt with, or a fleeting fantasy, was detrimental to your sexy lifestyle. If something makes you hot, act on it—you deserve to feel good. Don't let a chance to have a yummy O pass you by! Fueling your Mojo with these things should be almost second nature by now—keep it up!

✓ *Remember to tell yourself sexy self-love sayings*

By now, you should be really tuned in to your negative body banter habits. Now that you're more aware of them, you can catch them as they're happening and turn them around. When I catch myself heading into a negative zone, I clap my hands twice, and say out loud, *Enough!* And then I lay some positive banter on my gorgeous self. Sending affirmations to yourself on your phone or laptop (or with notes on a mirror or in a drawer) is another trick that will boost you up and keep you there. Messages can say something as simple as, *Hi, sexy!* or, *Have you had your dose of sexy satisfaction today, hot stuff?* Yes, it's sort of goofy, but that's part of the fun—you'll smile wide every time you come across a message, and right there, that's a boost!

✓ *Continue looking for visual stimulation*

Whether it's watching the way a man walks down the street, smelling his scent, or spotting a well-endowed carrot at the farmers' market, it's crucial to keep your senses open to those quick moments that encourage your inner lust. Use your cell phone to record verbal reports as you spot steamy stuff . . . then play them back whenever you're in the mood for a fun pick-me-up. You can also take photos or mini–video clips with your phone and view them at will. At your next weekly girlfriend group, everyone can make a pact that when they spot something hot they'll snap photos and e-mail them to the group or Tweet about it—anything from a hot guy to a seductive flower to a racy piece of lingerie you crave in a store to a sexy shot of yourself when you feel extra hot.

✓ *Keep pushing your limits*

Remember, your work doesn't stop at the end of this book. Continue to dig deeper, seek sexier, and fly higher! Revisit the list of sexy scenarios in Chapter 19 and tackle them one by one, including versions of the ones you didn't think were your cup of tea. Or combine ideas and craft your own steamy vignette. Sometimes you can surprise yourself with what you find pleasure in. Also, don't forget to communicate with your lover—a partner who has been along for your Mojo-awakening ride will certainly have some sexy ideas you can explore together. The same goes with your friends. The more Mojo mind melds, the better for everyone!

MY SECRET MOJO MAINTENANCE SPELL

As a last fun exercise, I'm going to share my sexy, spiritual love ritual with you. It's a final way to adore yourself, and it's a powerful representation of your metamorphosis into a sexy, fabulous woman with a fully fired-up Mojo. That fire has the power to deliver whatever you want into your life.

💜 **Take a day to think about the ten things you want in your ultimate sexy lifestyle.** Dig deep inside for this . . . Peel back the layers of what you need and desire. What do you crave emotionally? What kind of connections do you want with others (your friends, your partner, potential lovers, coworkers)? Write the ten things on a piece of paper.

💜 **Prepare for your ritual.** Pick a night where you have privacy—you need about an hour of uninterrupted "me time." Choose an outfit that makes you feel uniquely you, terribly sexy, totally confident. The outfit is important because it's symbolic of your commitment to the spell—so keep a part of it on during the whole ritual.

💜 **Create your environment.** You need lighting that feels a little bit cosmic—candles, lights on dim, and maybe even a colored lightbulb. (This is a spell, after all!) You need music that makes you feel totally connected with the universe. (What's the song that makes your heart swell in your chest when you hear it? That makes you know that all is right in the world?) You need a glass of wine or other libation that gets you a little tipsy and uninhibited. You need a perfume that makes you feel really sexy and that totally represents who you are.

💜 **Set your bed with your tools for the spell.** Have your perfume nearby. You'll need your piece of paper. Put out your favorite sex toys.

♥ Move around in the mirror to the music; get into the groove; feel happy. Get excited. You're arousing all the Mojo that you've built up inside.

♥ Head over to the bed and create an incredible sexy solo session. Really draw it out—don't just orgasm immediately—but build yourself up, take your time. As you're pleasuring yourself, think of the ten things, and think of how ecstatic you'll feel when they are part of your life. See yourself in total elation. Banish any guilt, any feelings that you don't deserve what you want.

♥ Then, have a mind-blowing orgasm . . . as if you were orgasming to save the planet, as if you're offering up your true Mojo and light as a gift to the universe. I'm talking big energy, so let it loose!

♥ Right after you orgasm, take your list and press it right up against your lady spot (yes, right against it) so that a bit of your love rubs off on the paper.

♥ Mist the paper (and yourself) with your signature scent, then stow the paper in a secret place.

♥ Thank yourself for doing something totally pure toward your own personal happiness and satisfaction in love and life. And see what happens!

Be sure to *support* your effort by tending to your Mojo in all the ways you've learned from this makeover. Keep doing the Big 5-O program, hone your dirty-talk skills, build an army of sex toys! Keep that heat cranked up!

IT'S INDEPENDENCE DAY!

Foxy lady,

I salute you. You've made it through the days and weeks of self-discovery, and allowed your gorgeous sexiness to bubble up and flow around all parts of your life. You triggered elation in ways you never thought you would. (And you liked it.) That's no small feat. Investing in yourself is a way to say, I love you to . . . you. You deserve the freedom, the confidence, the pleasure that you've brought to your world. I'm beyond proud and hope that you don't ever let the fires fade. I'm here for you from now on as your cheerleader. Keep on motivating that Mojo!

xoxo

Dana

Appendix

BECOME AN ADVOCATE FOR FEMALE MOJO!

Imagine if more and more women found their way to Mojo happiness and came to the gorgeous realization that they are powerfully in control of their desires. If more women really believed that they deserve a place at the top of the who-matters list in their own lives. With this makeover under your belt, you have what it takes to spread the sexy self-confidence magic to those around you. Invite new ladies into your weekly girls' night. Compliment people. Flirt innocently—it makes the flirt-ee feel as good as you do when you get their energy back.

Remember: With knowledge comes power, and sharing that power with other women in need will help to fuel the sexy revolution, creating sexy, satisfied, self-confident women all over the world! Check out www.bootyparlor.com for more info.

ABOUT BOOTY PARLOR

Booty Parlor, the beauty parlor for your love life, was conceived on the premise that confidence is the sexiest thing a woman can have.

We believe that every woman deserves to feel sexy, desirable, and satisfied. Our award-winning products are therefore specifically designed to boost a woman's sexy self-confidence and inspire her to create sexy experiences—inside and outside of the bedroom.

Founded in 2004 by married couple Charlie and Dana B. Myers, Booty Parlor products are sold in many of the world's leading boutiques and hotels, as well as by a network of Sexy Lifestyle Advisors, who deliver personalized sexy lifestyle consultations and shopping sessions at fabulous in-home Sexy Shopping Parties.

Acknowledgments

WORDS CAN'T FULLY EXPRESS MY GRATITUDE TO ALL THE people who helped make this book possible . . . but here's my best shot!

First, mega-thanks to my mom, Barbara. You set the example for feminine confidence, sparkling beauty, entrepreneurship, and pure love. I'm so very lucky to have you.

Dad, you raised me to be determined, hardworking, and to never, ever quit. You made sure I knew I could do anything I set my mind to, and then you helped me get there. Thank you!

To JD, I love you, bro. Who thought we'd ever do seminars together on weight loss and sex!

To the rest of my family, Chelsea, Rog and Lee, Seffie and Nick, and the rest of the gang. Your positivity and all-around support for Charlie and me has been, and continues to be, truly amazing. Big, big thanks.

To Eileen Cope, my incredible agent at Trident Media Group. You *got it* right away, and you made it happen. Charlie and I are endlessly grateful!

To Stephanie Meyers, my fabulous (and patient!) editor at HarperCollins. It's been a gorgeous collaboration—thank you so much for your insightful edits and for believing in the message of the Mojo Makeover.

To Mary Rose Almasi—you are the genius I was looking for all along! Our Mojo mind melds made it seem easy, huh? Thank you so much for your talent, humor, honesty, support, and deep understanding of the material. Together, we brought this makeover to a whole new level.

To Roger, thank you so much for your trust and support over the years.

To the BP team, it's because of you that our little dream has become the company it is today. We couldn't do it without you!

To all my Sexy Lifestyle Advisors, thank you for embracing our philosophy, our products, and the Mojo Makeover. I'm so excited to be your partner on this sexy revolution. Now, let's keep rocking!

To Naomi, Gia, Beth, Dara, Jane, Rosalie, Whitney, Summer, Cat, Gita, Suzette, Lisa, Colleen, Tess, Julia, Angela, Amy, Allison, and the rest of my Mojo ladies—thank you for being my Model citizens. I'm so grateful for your complete honesty and willingness to share your experiences with the women who will read this book. Your feedback and stories are what make this journey so rich—you made it a sisterhood.

To my girls—Meg, Dommie, Jenny, and Muffs. You're my best friends, and I simply couldn't live without your love! (And I adore the rest of you, too . . . Claudia, Kiki, T-Rex, Sara, Rizzo, Rena . . . xoxoxo!)

To Carly, I'm grateful for the kick-start.

To R, my little rock star. You were my silent partner on this adventure. It was the first of many, so get ready!

And to Charlie . . . You are the man behind the makeover! This book is as much yours as it is mine. Congratulations on it, love. As my husband, you light me up; you turn me on; you take the very best care of me. Your love makes everything possible. As my business partner, you constantly inspire me with your vision, your drive, your brilliant ideas, your tenacity. I'm forever crazy about you, forever grateful to you. There's nothing we can't do together.

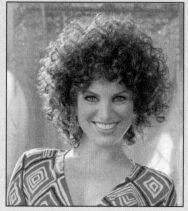

Dominick Guillemot

About the Author

As founder of Booty Parlor, America's premiere sexy beauty-and-lifestyle brand, Dana B. Myers has inspired thousands of women, from A-list celebrities to stay-at-home moms, to boost their sexy self-confidence and create sexier, more satisfying experiences, inside and outside of the bedroom.

Dana is an award-winning product developer, entrepreneur, and Sexy Lifestyle Expert who is regularly profiled in the media. Her line of Seductive Beauty Products and Bedroom Accessories is sold in many of the world's leading retail stores and hotels. Dana is also mentor to thousands of independent Sexy Lifestyle Advisors who represent Booty Parlor across the U.S.

Before starting Booty Parlor, Dana's first love was music. She is a classically trained concert pianist, and she graduated from the renowned music program at DePaul University in Chicago before earning a Master of Arts degree in music business from NYU.

Dana has always been the go-to girl for love and sex advice. With her Mojo Makeover program, her vision is to provide women with the tips, tricks, and advice they need to revamp their love lives, amp up their sex appeal, and boost their sexy self-confidence.

Dana lives in Los Angeles, California, with her husband and business partner, Charlie, and their son, Rocky.